Lunch IN FIVE

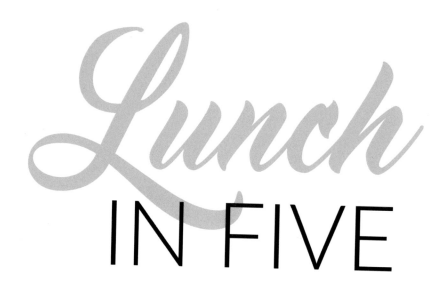

30 low-carb lunches

Up to **5** net carbs, **5** ingredients & **5** easy steps for every recipe

Vicky Ushakova and Rami Abramov

Table of Contents

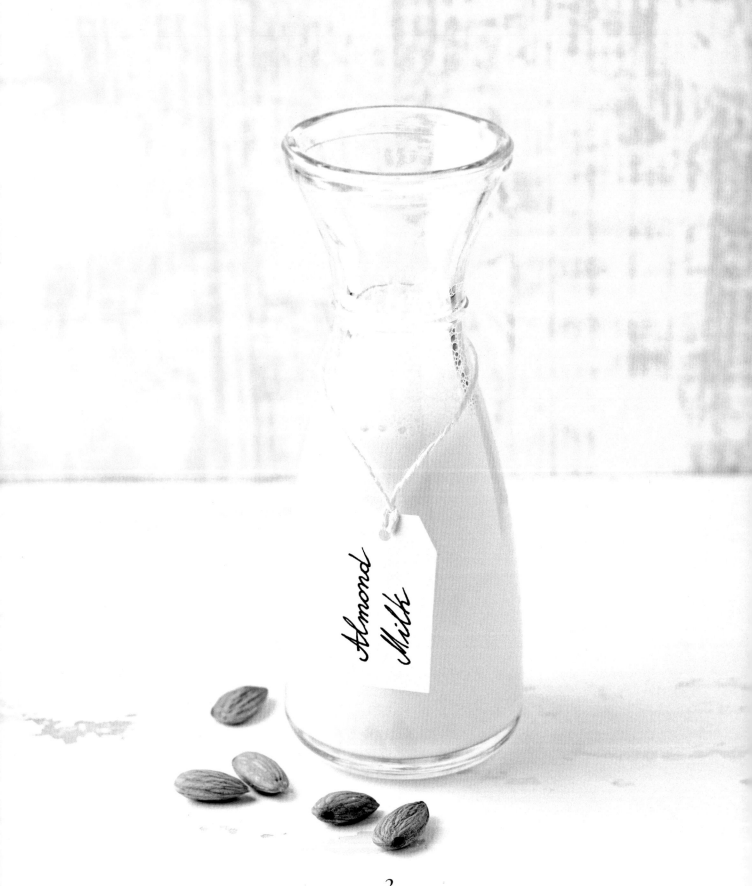

Disclaimer

Limit of Liability/Disclaimer of Warranty: Tasteaholics, Inc. is not a medical company or organization. Our books provide information in respect to healthy eating, nutrition and recipes and are intended for informational purposes only. We are not nutritionists or doctors and the information in this book and our website is not meant to be given as medical advice. We are two people sharing our success strategies and resources and encouraging you to do further research to see if they'll work for you too. Before starting any diet, you should always consult with your physician to rule out any health issues that could arise. Safety first, results second. Do not disregard professional medical advice or delay in seeking it because of this book.

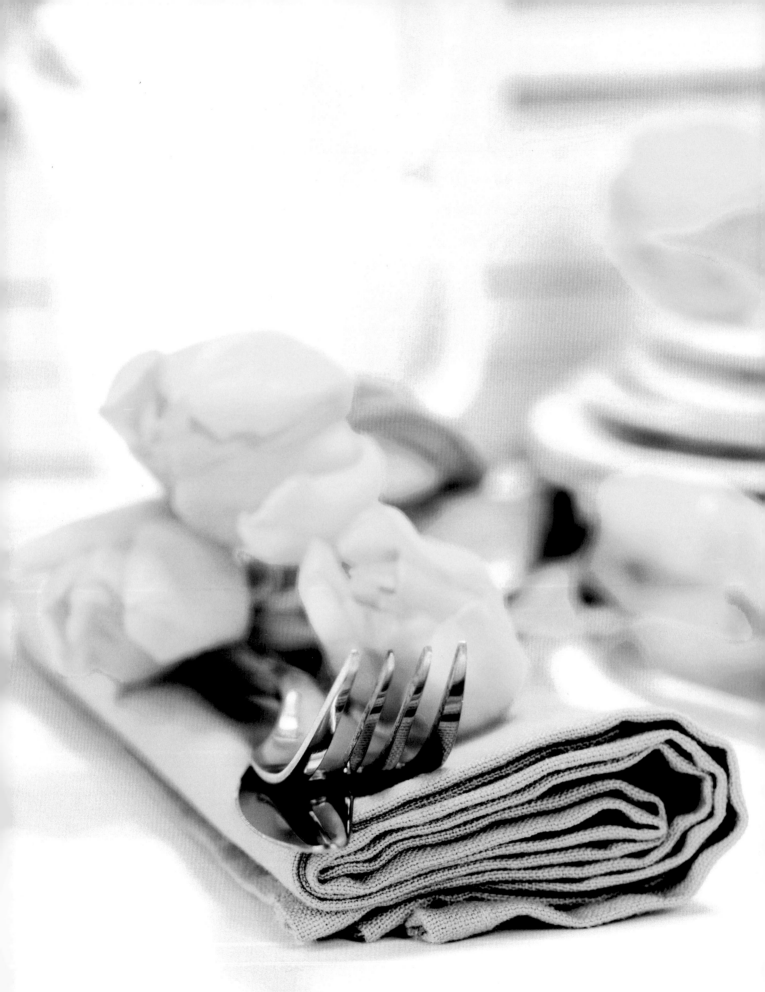

About This Book

This book was designed as a guide to help you kick start your ketogenic diet so you can lose weight, become healthy and have high energy levels every day.

Inside this book, you'll find the basics of the ketogenic diet, useful tips and delicious lunch recipes.

Each recipe is only 5 grams of net carbs or fewer and can be made with just 5 ingredients! There's nothing better than that.

Eating low-carb doesn't require cutting out wholesome, nutritious foods or sacrificing taste — ever. We hand selected each ingredient to not only serve a delicious purpose but provide nutritious benefits.

Enjoy 30 delicious and easy low-carb lunch recipes including crepes, salads, soups, stir fries, casseroles & curries that'll keep you full and excited for tomorrow's lunch.

Let's get started!

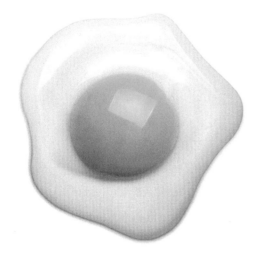

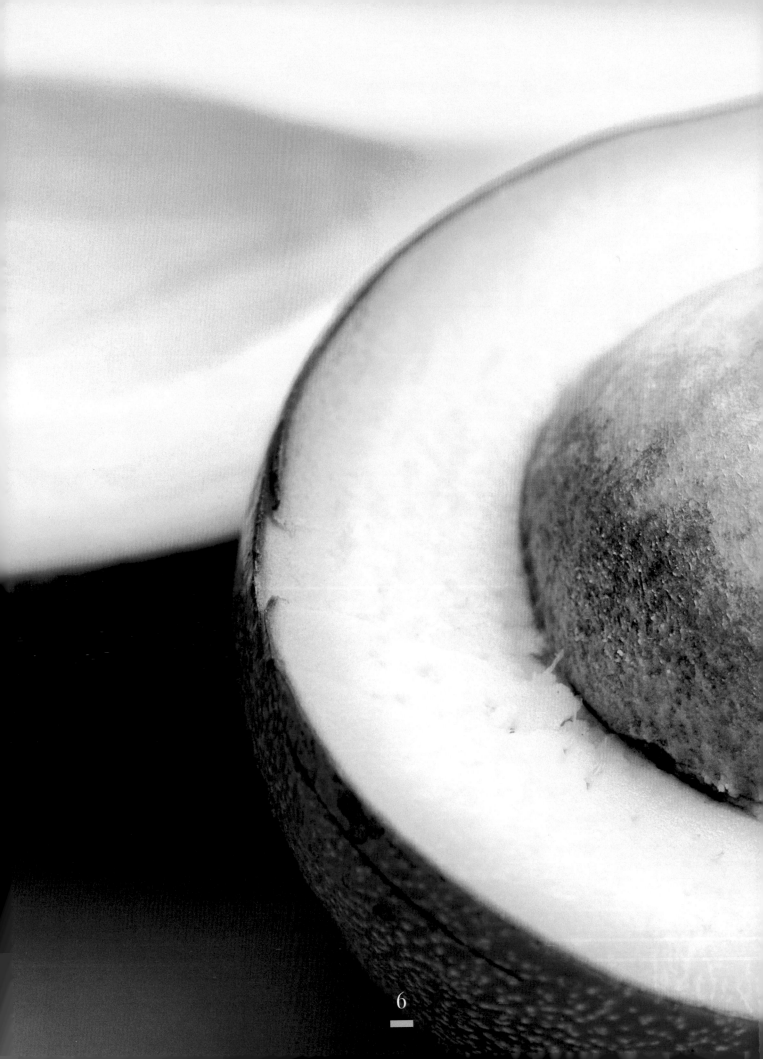

Keto 101

What Is Keto?

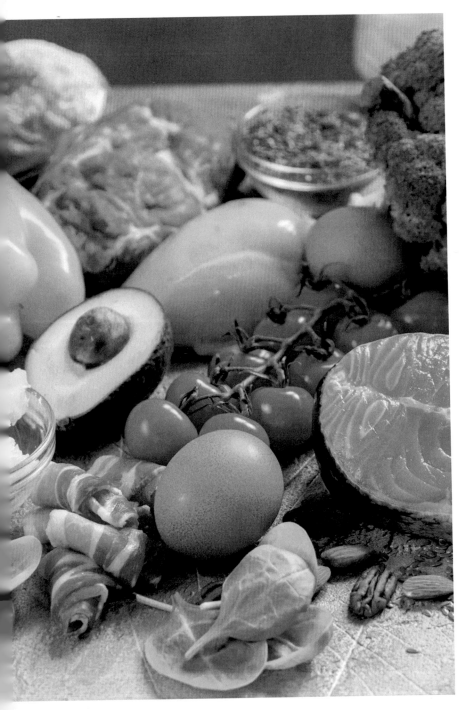

The Ketogenic Diet

The ketogenic (or keto) diet is a low-carbohydrate, high-fat diet. Maintaining this diet is a great tool for weight loss. More importantly, according to an increasing number of studies, it reduces risk factors for diabetes, heart diseases, stroke, Alzheimer's, epilepsy, and more.[1-6]

On the keto diet, your body enters a metabolic state called ketosis. While in ketosis your body is using ketone bodies for energy instead of glucose. Ketone bodies are derived from fat and are a much more stable, steady source of energy than glucose, which is derived from carbohydrates.

Entering ketosis usually takes anywhere from 3 days to a week. Once you're in ketosis, you'll be using fat for energy, instead of carbs. This includes the fat you eat and stored body fat.

While eating low-carb, you'll lose weight easier, feel satiated longer and enjoy consistent energy levels throughout your day.

Testing for Ketosis

You can test yourself to see whether you've entered ketosis just a few days after you've begun the keto diet! Use a *ketone urine test strip* and it will tell you the level of ketone bodies in your urine. If the concentration is high enough and the test strip shows any hue of purple, you've successfully entered ketosis!

The strips take only a few seconds to show results and are the fastest and most affordable way to check whether you're in ketosis.

Visit tasteaholics.com/strips and get a bottle of 100 test strips.

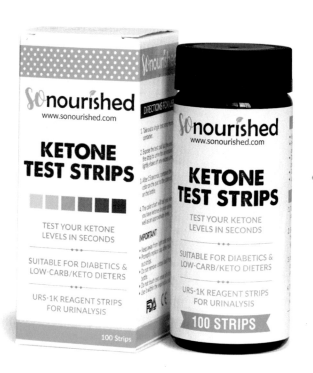

The Truth About Fat

You may be thinking, "but eating a lot of fat is bad!" The truth is, dozens of studies and meta studies with over 900,000 subjects have arrived at similar conclusions: eating saturated and monounsaturated fats have no effects on heart disease risks.[7,8]

Most fats are good and are essential to our health. Fats (fatty acids) and protein (amino acids) are essential for survival.

> **There is no such thing as an essential carbohydrate.**

Fats are the most efficient form of energy and each gram contains more than double the energy in a gram of protein or carbohydrates (more on that later).

The keto diet promotes eating fresh, whole foods like meat, fish, veggies, and healthy fats and oils as well as greatly reducing processed and chemically treated foods the Standard American Diet (SAD) has so long encouraged.

It's a diet that you can sustain long-term and enjoy. What's not to enjoy about bacon and eggs in the morning?

Calories & Macro-nutrients

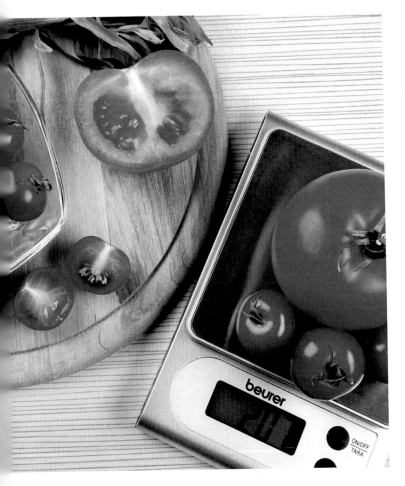

How Calories Work

A calorie is a unit of energy. When something contains 100 calories, it describes how much energy your body could get from consuming it. Calorie consumption dictates weight gain/loss.

If you burn an average of 1,800 calories and eat 2,000 calories per day, you will gain weight.

If you do light exercise that burns an extra 300 calories per day, you'll burn 2,100 calories per day, putting you at a deficit of 100 calories. Simply by eating at a deficit, you will lose weight because your body will tap into stored resources for the remaining energy it needs.

That being said, it's important to get the right balance of macronutrients every day so your body has the energy it needs.

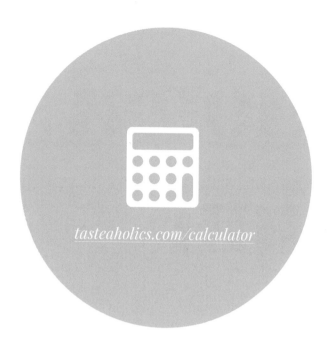

What Are Macronutrients?

Macronutrients (macros) are molecules that our bodies use to create energy for themselves – primarily fat, protein and carbs. They are found in all food and are measured in grams (g) on nutrition labels.

- **Fat** provides 9 calories per gram
- **Protein** provides 4 calories per gram
- **Carbs** provide 4 calories per gram

Learn more at tasteaholics.com/macros.

Net Carbs

Most low-carb recipes write net carbs when displaying their macros. Net carbs are total carbs minus dietary fiber and sugar alcohols. Our bodies can't break them down into glucose so they don't count toward your total carb count.

Note: *Dietary fiber can be listed as soluble or insoluble.*

How Much Should You Eat?

On a keto diet, about 65 to 75 percent of the calories you consume daily should come from fat. About 20 to 30 percent should come from protein. The remaining 5 percent or so should come from carbohydrates.

Use our keto calculator to figure out exactly how many calories and macros you should be eating every day!

It will ask for basic information including your weight, activity levels and goals and instantly provide you with the total calories and grams of fat, protein and carbs that you should be eating each day.

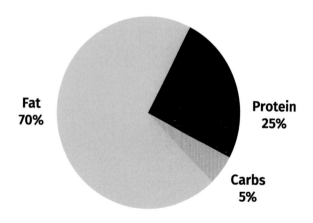

Note: *The calculator should be used as a general guideline. The results are based on your inputs and variables such as body fat percentage and basal metabolic rate are difficult to estimate correctly.*

A Nutritional Revolution

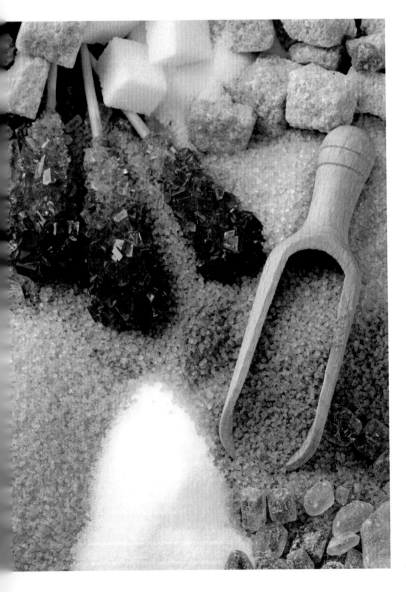

Carbs: What Exactly Are They?

Carbohydrates (carbs) are found in things like starches, grains and foods high in sugar. This includes, but isn't limited to, bread, flour, rice, pasta, beans, potatoes, sugar, syrup, cereals, fruits, bagels and soda.

Carbs are broken down into glucose (a type of sugar) in our bodies for energy. Eating any kinds of carbs spikes blood sugar levels. The spike may happen faster or slower depending on the type of carb (based on the glycemic index), but the spike will still happen.

Blood sugar spikes cause strong insulin releases to combat the spikes. Constant insulin releases result in fat storage and insulin resistance. After many years, this cycle can lead to prediabetes, metabolic syndrome and even type 2 diabetes.[9]

In a world full of sugar, cereal, pasta, burgers, French fries and large sodas, you can see how carbs can easily be overconsumed.

Where We Are Today

According to the 2014 report by the Centers for Disease Control and Prevention (CDC), more than 1 in 3 adults in the U.S. (86 million people) have prediabetes, a condition in which blood glucose is always high and commonly leads to type 2 diabetes and many other medical problems.[10]

Today, almost 1 in 10 people in the U.S. have type 2 diabetes compared to almost 1 in 40 in 1980.

Fat has been blamed as the bad guy and carbohydrates have been considered crucial and healthy. Companies have been creating low-fat and fat-free, chemical-laden alternatives of nearly every type of food in existence, yet diabetes and heart disease rates are still increasing.

Fat Is Making a Comeback

Hundreds of studies have been conducted in the past ten years which have been corroborating the same data: that eating healthy fats is not detrimental to health and is, in fact, more beneficial than eating a diet high in carbohydrates.

We're starting to understand that carbs in large quantities are much more harmful than previously thought, while most fats are healthy and essential.

The nutritional landscape is changing. Low-carb and similar dietary groups are growing and a nutritional revolution is beginning. We are beginning to realize the detrimental effects of our relationship with excess sugar and carbs.

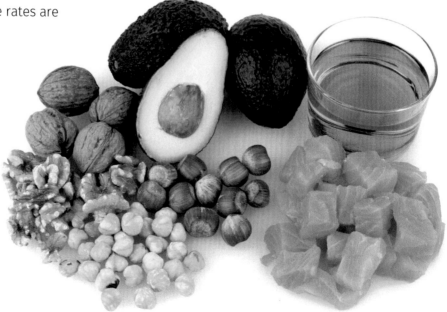

The Basics: Benefits of Going Keto

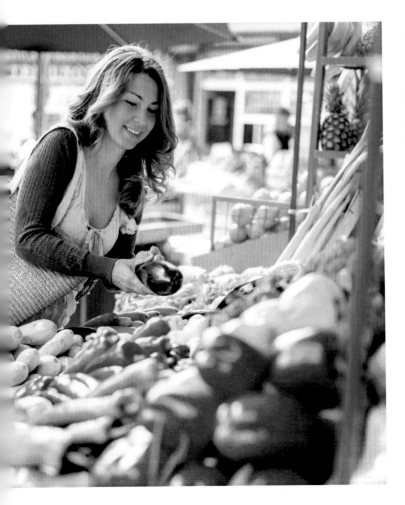

Long-Term Benefits

Studies consistently show that those who eat a low-carb, high-fat diet rather than a high-carb, low-fat diet:

- Lose more weight and body fat[11–17]

- Have better levels of good cholesterol (HDL and large LDL)[18,19]

- Have reduced blood sugar and insulin resistance (commonly reversing prediabetes and type 2 diabetes)[20,21]

- Experience a decrease in appetite[22]

- Have reduced triglyceride levels (fat molecules in the blood that cause heart disease)[19,23]

- Have significant reductions in blood pressure, leading to a reduction in heart disease and stroke[24]

Day-To-Day Benefits

The keto diet doesn't only provide long-term benefits! When you're on keto, you can expect to:

- Lose body fat
- Have stable energy levels during the day
- Stay satiated after meals longer, with less snacking and overeating

Longer satiation and consistent energy levels are due to the majority of calories coming from fat, which is slower to digest and calorically denser.

Eating low-carb also eliminates blood glucose spikes and crashes. You won't have sudden blood sugar drops leaving you feeling weak and disoriented.

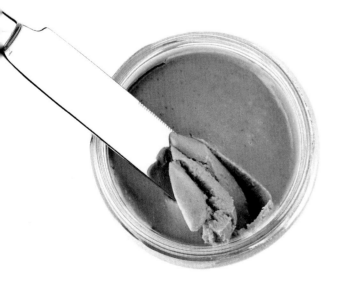

Entering Ketosis

The keto diet's main goal is to keep you in nutritional ketosis all the time. If you're just getting started with your keto diet, you should eat up to 25 grams of carbs per day.

Once you're in ketosis for long enough (about 4 to 8 weeks), you become keto-adapted, or fat-adapted. This is when your glycogen stores in muscles and liver are depleted, you carry less water weight, muscle endurance increases and your overall energy levels are higher.

Once keto-adapted, you can usually eat ≈50 grams of net carbs a day to maintain ketosis.

Type 1 Diabetes & Ketoacidosis

If you have type 1 diabetes, consult with your doctor before starting a keto diet. Diabetic ketoacidosis (DKA) is a dangerous condition that can occur if you have type 1 diabetes due to a shortage of insulin.

Steering Clear of the Keto Flu

What Is the Keto Flu?

The keto flu happens commonly to keto dieters due to low levels of sodium and electrolytes and has flu-like symptoms including:

- Fatigue
- Headaches
- Cough
- Sniffles
- Irritability
- Nausea

It's important to note that this isn't the real flu! It's called keto flu due to similar symptoms but it is not at all contagious and doesn't actually involve a virus.

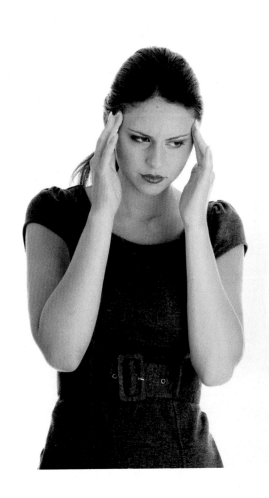

Why Does It Happen?

The main cause of keto flu is your body lacking electrolytes, especially sodium. When starting keto, you cut out lots of processed foods and eat more whole, natural foods. Although this is great, it causes a sudden drop in sodium intake.

> **The keto flu can be avoided by consuming enough electrolytes, especially sodium.**

In addition, reducing carbs reduces insulin levels, which reduces sodium stored by kidneys.[25]

Between your reduced sodium intake and stored sodium flushed by your kidneys, you end up being low on sodium and other electrolytes.

Ending the Keto Flu

The best way to avoid or end the keto flu is to add more sodium and electrolytes to your diet. Here are the most effective (and tasty) ways to get more sodium:

- Adding more salt to your food
- Drinking soup broth
- Eating plenty of salty foods like bacon and pickled vegetables

Try to eat more sodium as you start the keto diet to prevent the keto flu entirely. If you do catch it, just remember that it'll go away quickly and you'll emerge a fat-burning machine!

Note: *For more information about the keto flu, read our full guide at tasteaholics.com/keto-flu.*

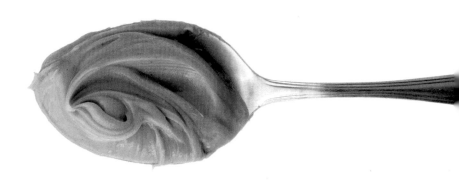

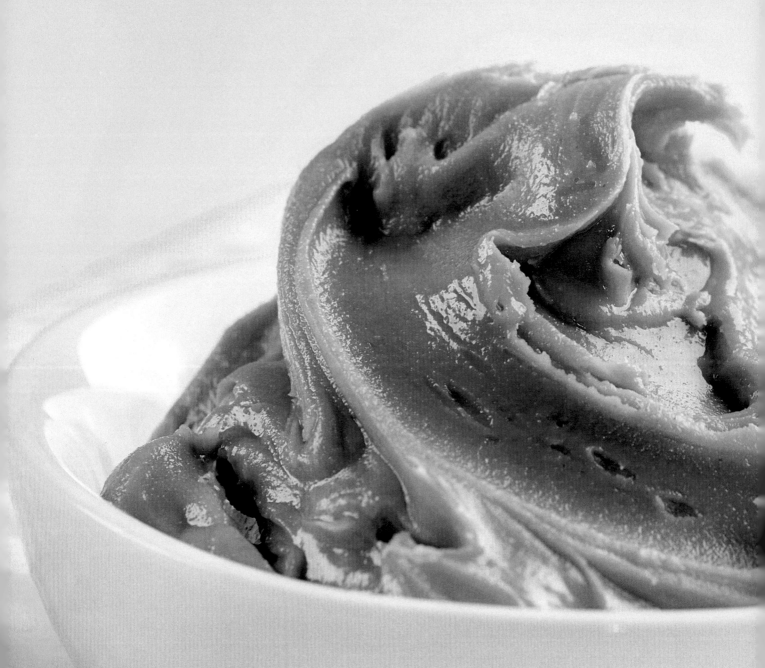

Starting Keto

Part 1 — Out with the Old

Having tempting, unhealthy foods in your home is one of the biggest reasons for failure when starting any diet.

To maximize your chances of success, you need to remove as many triggers as you can. This crucial step will help prevent moments of weakness from ruining all your hard work.

If you aren't living alone, make sure to discuss with your family or housemates before throwing anything out. If some items are simply not yours to throw out, try to compromise and agree on a special location so you can keep them out of sight and out of mind.

Once your home is free of temptation, eating low-carb is far less difficult and success is that much easier.

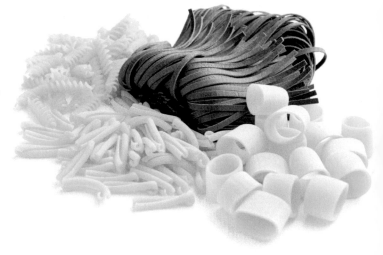

Starches and Grains

Get rid of all cereal, pasta, bread, rice, potatoes, corn, oats, quinoa, flour, bagels, rolls, croissants and wraps.

All Sugary Things

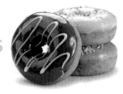

Throw away and forget all refined sugar, fruit juices, desserts, fountain drinks, milk chocolate, pastries, candy bars, etc.

Legumes

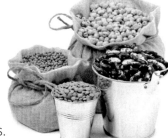

Discard or donate any beans, peas, and lentils.

Vegetable & Seed Oils

Stop using any vegetable oils and seed oils like sunflower, safflower, soybean, canola, corn and grapeseed oil. Get rid of trans fats like margarine.

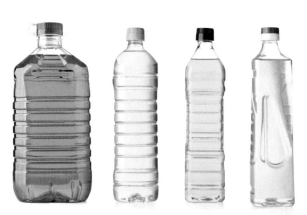

Read Nutrition Labels

Check the nutrition labels on all your products to see if they're high in carbs. There are hidden carbs in the unlikeliest of places (like ketchup and canned soups). Try to avoid buying products with dozens of incomprehensible ingredients. Less is usually healthier.

For example:

Deli ham can have 2 or 3 grams of sugar per slice as well as many added preservatives and nitrites!

Always check the serving sizes against the carb counts. Manufacturers can sometimes recommend inconceivably small serving sizes to seemingly reduce calorie and carb numbers.

At first glance, something may be low in carbs, but a quick comparison to the serving size can reveal the product is mostly sugar. Be diligent!

Nutrition Facts

Serving Size 1 Cup (53g/1.9 oz.)
Servings Per Container About 8

Amount Per Serving

Calories 190	Calories from Fat 25
	% Daily Value*
Total Fat 3g	5%
Saturated Fat 0g	0%
Trans Fat 0g	
Cholesterol 0mg	0%
Sodium 100mg	4%
Potassium 300mg	9%
Total Carbohydrate 37g	12%
Dietary Fiber 8g	32%
Soluble Fiber	
Insoluble Fibe	
Sugars 13g	
Protein 9g	14%
Vitamin A 0%	C 0%

Part 2 — In with the New!

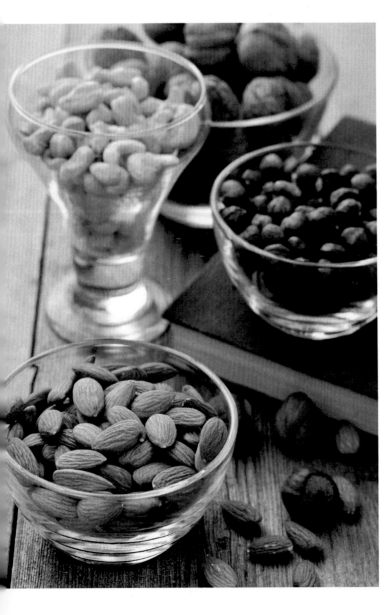

Now that you've cleaned out everything you don't need, it's time to restock your pantry and fridge with delicious and wholesome, keto-friendly foods that will help you lose weight, become healthier, and feel amazing!

General Products to Have

With these basics in your home, you'll always be ready to make healthy, keto-friendly meals.

- Lots of water, coffee, and unsweetened tea
- Stevia and erythritol (sweeteners)
- Condiments like mayonnaise, mustard, pesto, and sriracha
- Broths (beef, chicken, bone)
- Pickles and other fermented foods
- Seeds and nuts (chia seeds, flaxseeds, pecans, almonds, walnuts, macadamias, etc.)

Meat, Fish & Eggs

Just about every type of fresh meat and fish is good for keto including beef, chicken, lamb, pork, salmon, tuna, etc. Eat grass-fed and/or organic meat and wild-caught fish whenever possible.

Eat as many eggs as you like, preferably organic from free-range chickens.

Vegetables

Eat plenty of non-starchy veggies including asparagus, mushrooms, broccoli, cucumber, lettuce, onions, peppers, cauliflower, tomatoes, garlic, Brussels sprouts and zucchini.

Dairy

You can eat full-fat dairy like sour cream, heavy (whipping) cream, butter, cheeses and unsweetened yogurt.

Although not dairy, unsweetened almond milk and coconut milk are both good milk substitutes.

Stay away from regular milk, skim milk and sweetened yogurts because they contain a lot of sugar. Avoid all fat-free and low-fat dairy products.

Oils and Fats

Olive oil, avocado oil, butter and bacon fat are great for cooking and consuming. Avocado oil is best for searing due to its very high smoke point (520°F).

Fruits

Berries like strawberries, blueberries, raspberries, etc. are allowed in small amounts. Avocados are great because they're low-carb and very high in fat!

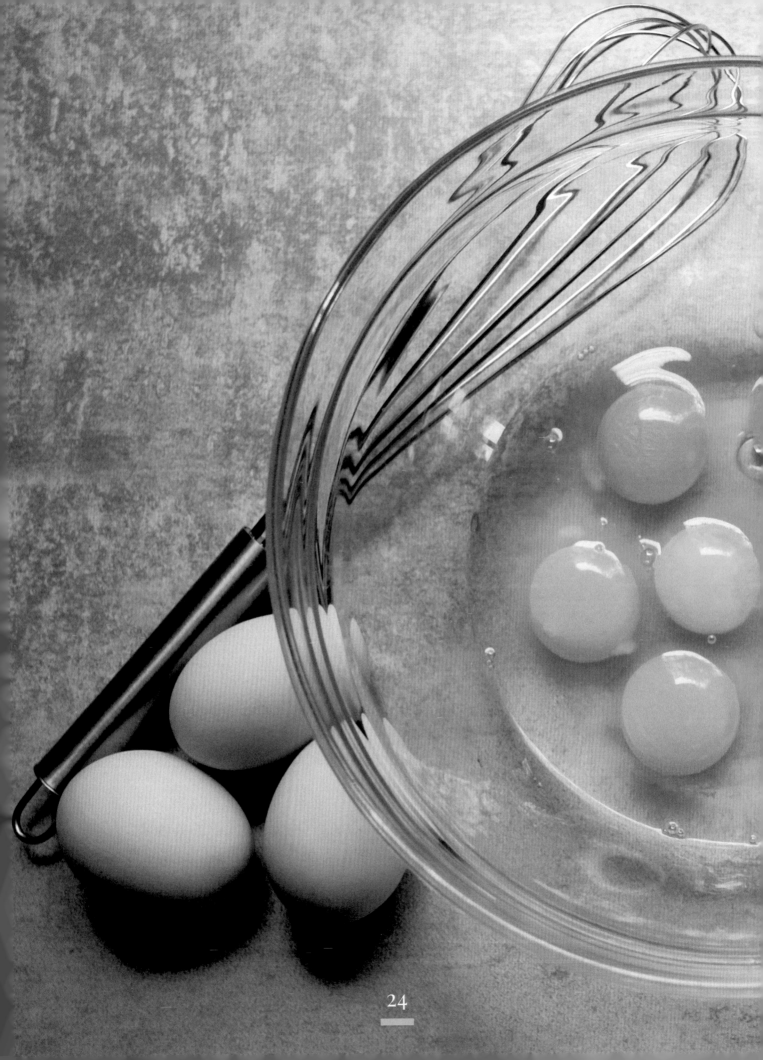

Recipes

Notes

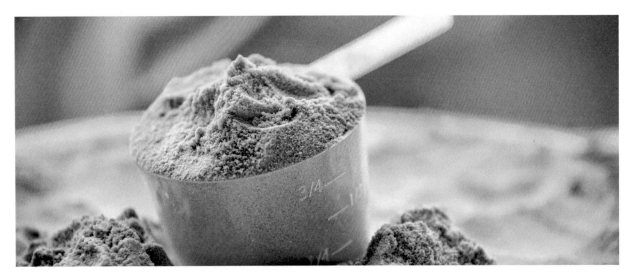

- We use large eggs in all our recipes. If yours are a different size, know that this will affect the nutrition slightly and perhaps the results.

- Use the most natural peanut and almond butter you can. The ingredients listed should be, at most, 2 ingredients long.

- If you don't have stevia, feel free to substitute your favorite sugar-free sweetener like erythritol, xylitol, Splenda, etc. Add a little at a time and work your way up to taste.
  - You can order erythritol online by visiting tasteaholics.com/erythritol.

- The mozzarella cheese in each recipe is a low-moisture, part-skim, shredded mozzarella cheese; not fresh mozzarella.

- Most recipes make 2 servings unless otherwise stated. The nutrition facts listed are per 1 serving.

- If you see the abbreviation "SF" it is short for "sugar-free".
  - For example, "SF Maple Syrup" means we used *Walden Farms* or *Sukrin Gold* syrup, both of which are sugar-free brands.

- If you're not a fan of spicy foods, feel free to leave out ingredients like jalapeño peppers, hot sauce, red pepper flakes, etc.

- The marinara sauce we use in all our recipes is of the brand *Rao's Homemade Sauces*. They are a low-sugar or no sugar added tomato sauce maker which can be found in many supermarkets. You can also choose to make your own from scratch or use any low-sugar tomato sauce you have on hand.

- A food scale is a must if you're counting calories and macros. Many of our ingredients are listed by weight to provide accurate nutritional data.

Low-Carb Friendly Seasonings

The following herbs and spices may be used in any of our recipes should you wish to add them.

They are all low-carb though we suggest limiting them to under a tablespoon to stay within your daily goals. It's more than enough to add their delicious flavors to your dishes without putting you over your carb limit!

☐ Salt
☐ Pepper
☐ Paprika
☐ Cayenne
☐ Thyme
☐ Basil
☐ Oregano
☐ Parsley
☐ Rosemary
☐ Tarragon
☐ Sage
☐ Cumin
☐ Red pepper flakes
☐ Sesame seeds

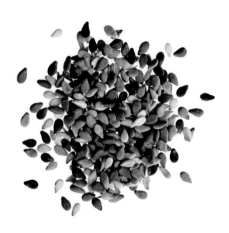

Savory French Crepe'wiches

We all know fruity, chocolatey crepes, but have you ever tried savory ones? You'll never look at crepes the same way again!

Nutrition

450 calories per serving | Makes 2 servings

34 grams of fat

32 grams of protein

2 grams of net carbs

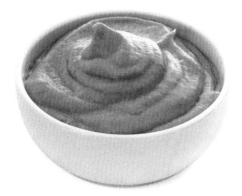

Ingredients

- 2 large eggs
- 2 oz. cream cheese
- 4 oz. cheddar cheese, shredded or sliced
- 4 oz. deli ham, sliced
- 1 tbsp. Dijon mustard

Instructions

1. Whisk the eggs and cream cheese together until smooth.
2. Add ¼ of the batter onto a very hot, lightly oiled frying pan. Spread quickly and thinly to reach the edges of the pan. Cook for 2 minutes, flip and cook the other side for 2 minutes. Repeat 3 more times until all the batter is cooked.
3. Add 1 oz. of cheddar, 1 oz. of ham and 1 teaspoon of Dijon mustard per crepe. Fold crepes to enclose the fillings and fry on the folded side for 20 seconds to seal it all in.
4. Cut diagonally and serve 4 triangles per serving.

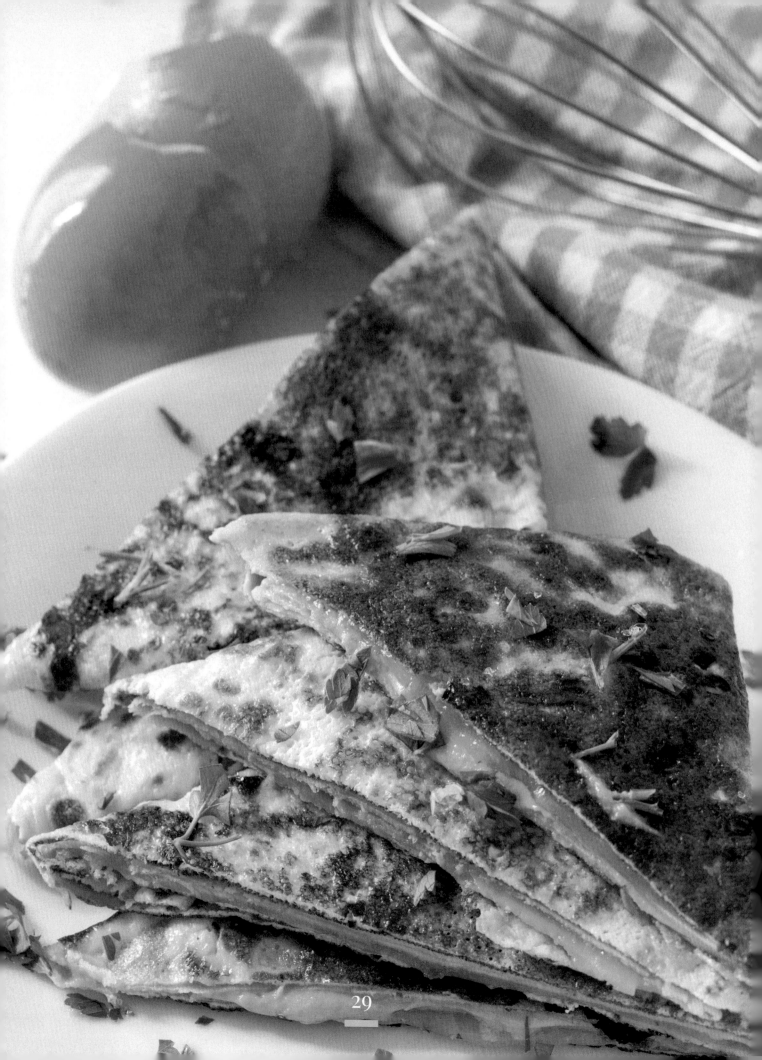

Asian Beef Slaw

Just because there's only 5 ingredients, doesn't mean this slaw is low on flavor. Juicy ground beef and tender veggies make a perfect combination.

Nutrition

480 calories per serving | Makes 4 servings

- 26 grams of fat
- 48 grams of protein
- 5 grams of net carbs

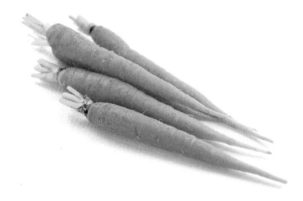

⏱ **Prep Time: 5 mins | Cook Time: 20 mins**

Ingredients

- 1 medium carrot
- 1 small green cabbage
- 1 lb. ground beef
- 2 tbsp. soy sauce
- 1 stalk green onion

Instructions

1. Shred the carrot and small cabbage.
2. Add the ground beef to a large frying pan or wok and break it up with a wooden spoon until very fine. Cook until browned.
3. Once browned, about 5–10 minutes, add in the shredded carrot, cabbage, soy sauce, and salt and pepper to taste. Toss well and cook for 5 minutes or until the cabbage has wilted.
4. Serve with chopped green onion and enjoy!

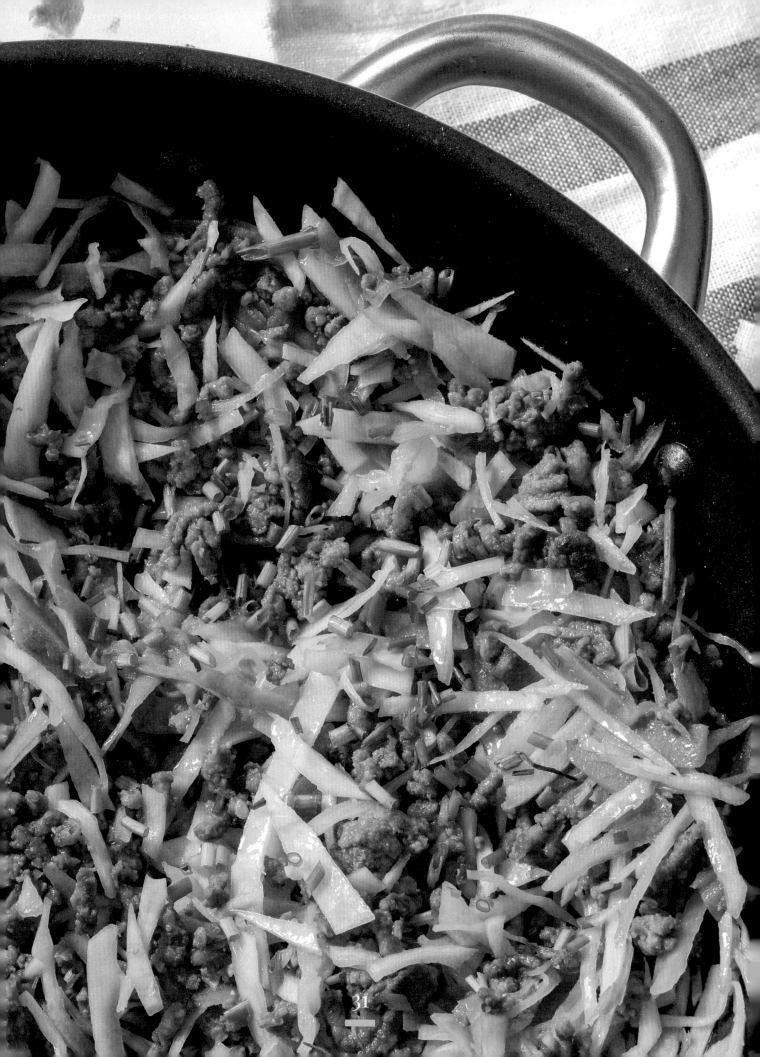

Coconut Chicken Curry

Coconut cream adds moisture and sweetness to this simple chicken curry. It makes for a great, high-fat lunch with some fresh green beans!

Nutrition

325 calories per serving | Makes 4 servings

▌ 16 grams of fat

▌ 38 grams of protein

▌ 5 grams of net carbs

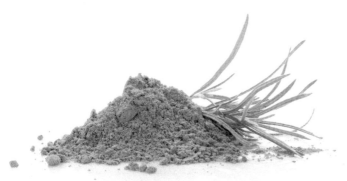

🕐 **Prep Time: 10 mins | Cook Time: 40 mins**

Ingredients

- ½ white onion, diced
- 24 oz. boneless skinless chicken thighs
- 14 oz. unsweetened canned coconut milk
- 2 cups green beans
- 1 tbsp. curry powder

Instructions

1. In an oiled pan on medium heat, cook onions until translucent, then take them off the pan.
2. Turn the heat up to high and once the pan is very hot, sear the chicken thighs for 3-5 minutes on each side. Then shred them using two forks or meat-shredding claws.
3. Combine shredded chicken, onion, coconut milk, chopped green beans, curry powder, salt and pepper in the pan and simmer on low for 20 minutes. The chicken should be fully cooked through and the green beans tender. Enjoy!

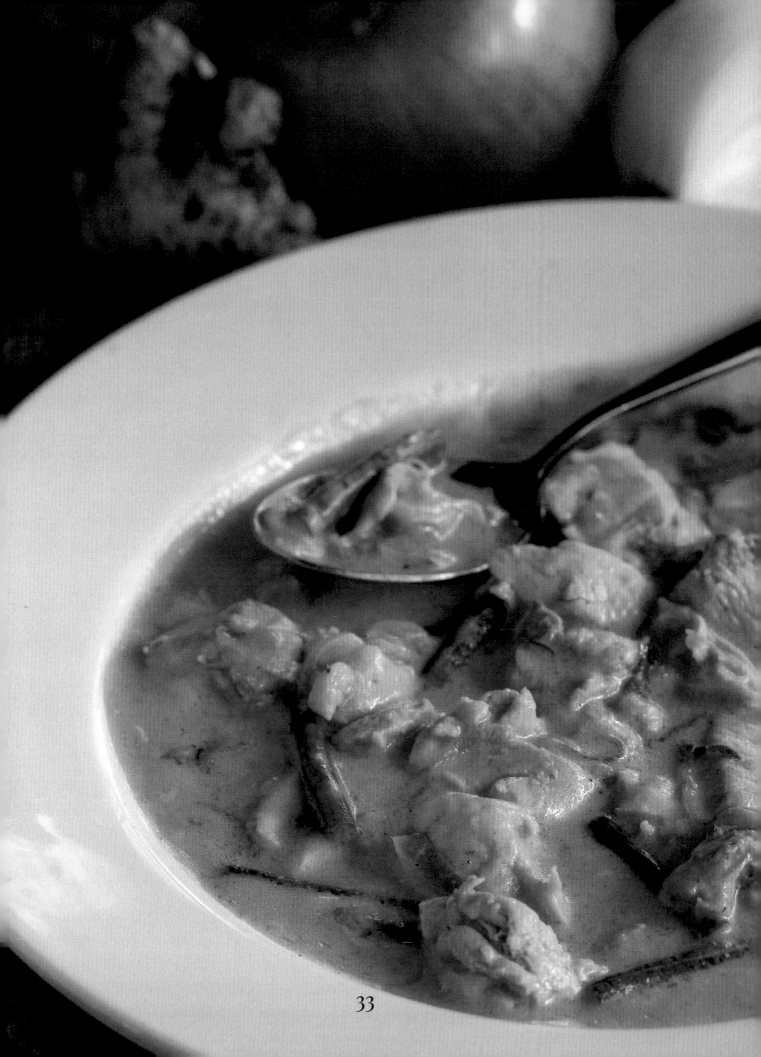

Miracle Spaghetti Bolognese

Saucy *Miracle Noodles* make this a healthy, light lunch with tons of flavor. Tiny, meaty chunks make this dish all about the fun noodles.

Nutrition

345 calories per serving | Makes 2 servings

| 24 grams of fat
| 27 grams of protein
| 3.5 grams of net carbs

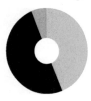

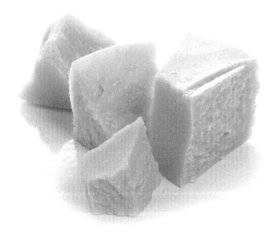

Ingredients

- 1 bag *Miracle Noodle* Spaghetti
- 1 lb. ground beef
- 2 cups marinara sauce
- 1 tsp. dried basil
- ½ cup shredded or shaved Parmesan cheese

Instructions

1. Prepare the *Miracle Noodle* Spaghetti according to the package instructions.
2. In a hot, oiled pan, brown the ground beef. Once it has almost fully cooked, add in the marinara sauce and simmer for 5 minutes.
3. Stir in the Miracle Spaghetti and season with salt, pepper and dried basil.
4. Serve topped with Parmesan.

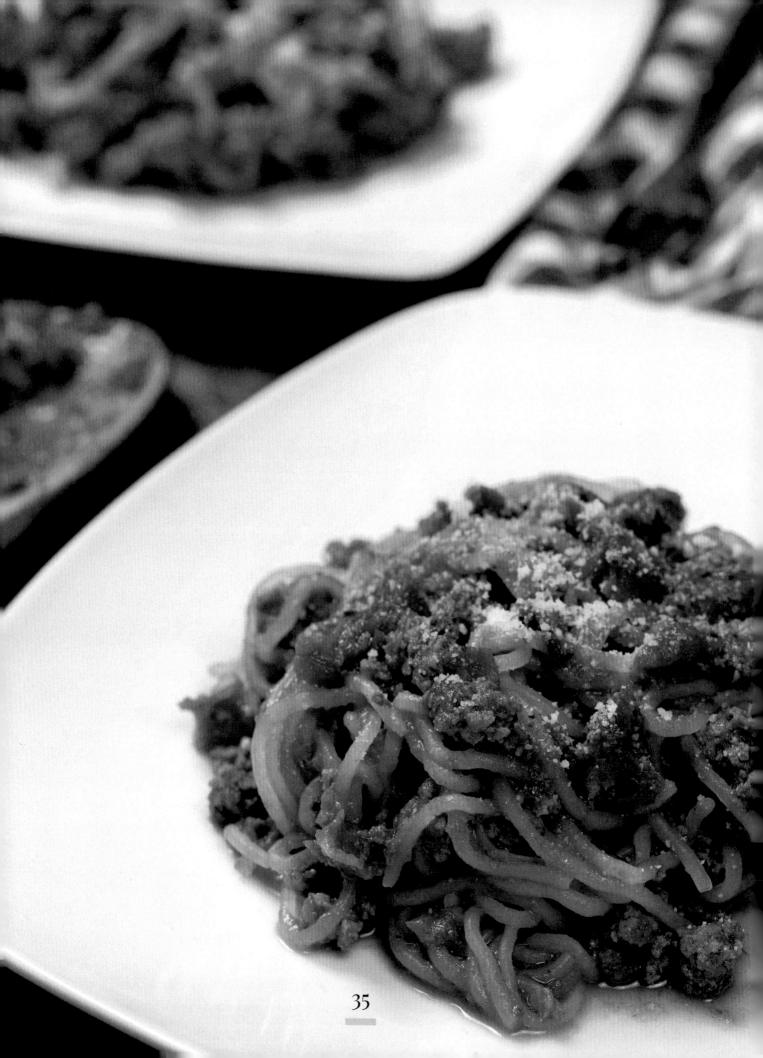

Classic Deviled Eggs

Eggs are so versatile! Take your basic boiled egg and turn it into a culinary masterpiece with the addition of a few key ingredients.

Nutrition

400 calories per serving | Makes 4 servings

- 34 grams of fat
- 19 grams of protein
- 2 grams of net carbs

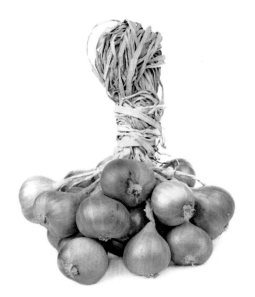

⏱ **Prep Time: 15 mins | Cook Time: 10 mins**

Ingredients

- 12 large eggs
- 1 shallot, finely diced
- 1 tbsp. Dijon mustard
- ½ cup mayonnaise
- 1 lime, juiced

Instructions

1. Set a pot of water to boil and lower your eggs in gently using a spoon. Let them boil for 10 minutes.
2. Peel and halve the boiled eggs, scooping the yolks out into a large mixing bowl. Set aside the whites.
3. Add in the shallots, mustard, mayonnaise, lime juice, salt and pepper into the egg yolks. Mash until smooth.
4. Spoon the egg yolk mixture back into the egg whites and serve chilled.

Tip: *Use a piping bag to pipe out the egg yolks for a more beautiful presentation!*

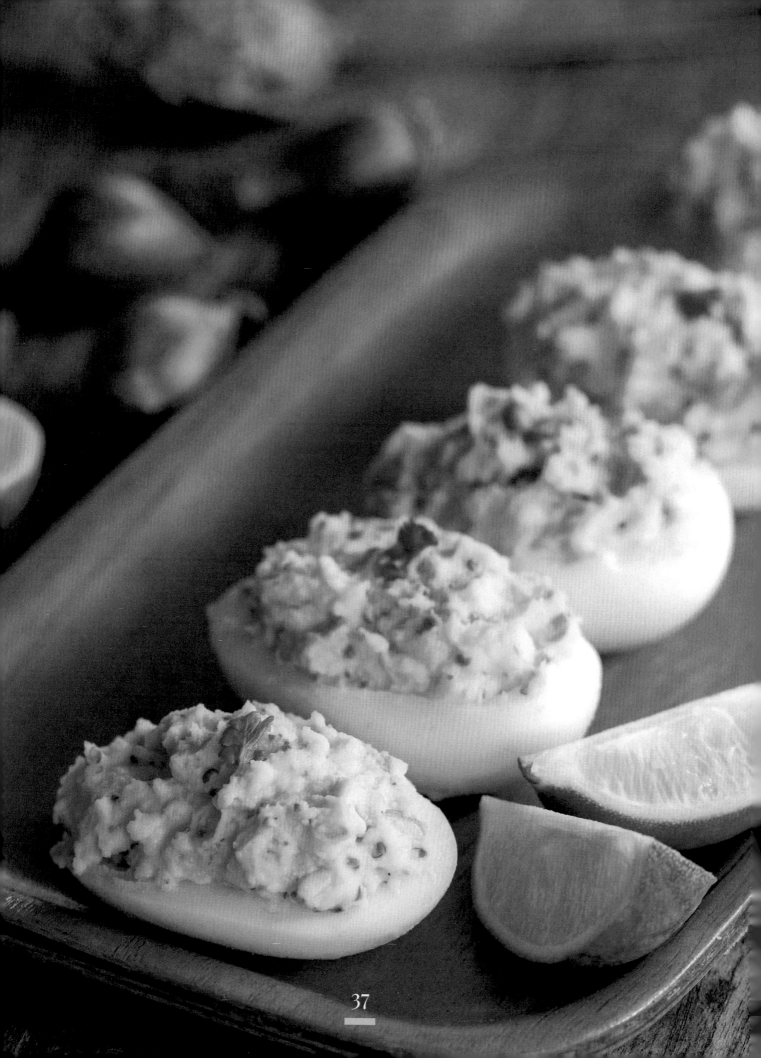

Jalapeño Chicken Casserole

A little spice and a whole lot of flavor will keep your friends and family coming back for more with this delicious jalapeño chicken casserole.

Nutrition

610 calories per serving | Makes 4 servings

47 grams of fat

44 grams of protein

5 grams of net carbs

Ingredients

- 1 lb. boneless skinless chicken thighs
- 3 cups broccoli florets
- ½ cup mayonnaise
- 2 ½ cups cheddar cheese, grated
- 1 fresh jalapeño, sliced

Instructions

1. Fry the chicken thighs in a well-oiled pan on medium heat until cooked. Shred them with 2 forks or meat-shredding claws.
2. Chop the broccoli florets and combine them with the chicken, mayonnaise, 2 cups of cheddar, and salt and pepper in a 9×13″ casserole dish. Bake for 25 minutes at 350°F.
3. In last 5 minutes of baking, top with the remaining cheddar and jalapeño slices.

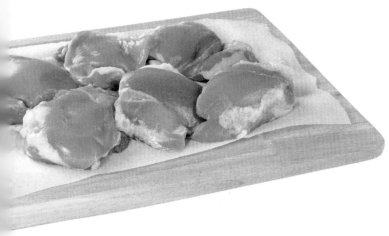

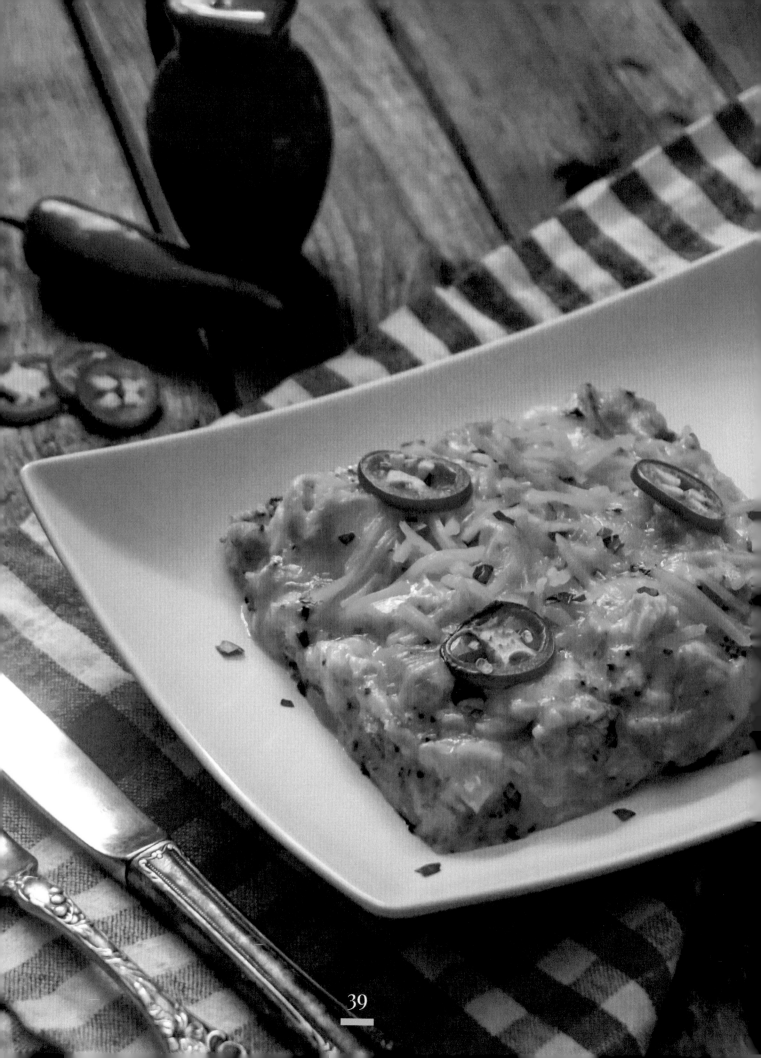

Cauliflower Stir-Fried Rice

Everyone loves Chinese food leftovers but not the carbs and calories! Cauliflower rice is here to make things low-carb and even more delicious.

Nutrition

420 calories per serving | Makes 2 servings

- 20 grams of fat
- 52 grams of protein
- 5 grams of net carbs

Ingredients

- 1 lb. boneless skinless chicken thighs, cubed
- 300 grams cauliflower florets
- 2 tbsp. unsalted butter
- 50 grams carrot, grated
- 50 grams broccoli, diced

Instructions

1. Add the cubed chicken to an oiled wok or deep skillet and fry on medium-high heat for 5 minutes or until almost fully cooked.
2. Meanwhile, pulse the cauliflower florets in a food processor until they resemble rice.
3. Add the riced cauliflower, butter, carrot and broccoli to the wok and fry for an additional 5–8 minutes, stirring continuously.
4. Season generously with salt and pepper and serve.

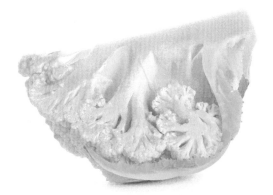

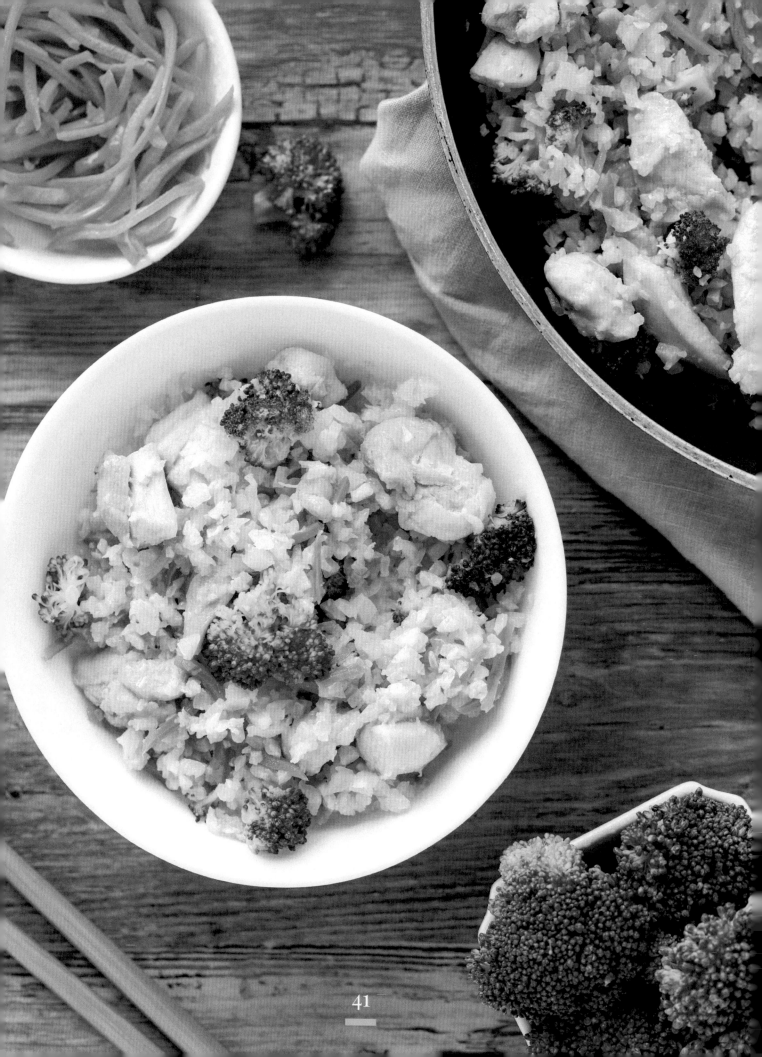

Cheesy Tuna Melt

Quick and tasty, our tuna melt is a favorite and an important staple in a keto diet. Nothing beats the speed and simplicity of this recipe.

Nutrition

482 calories per serving | Makes 2 servings

- 37 grams of fat
- 31 grams of protein
- 4 grams of net carbs

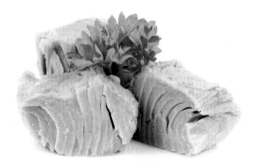

🕐 **Prep Time: 10 mins | Cook Time: 10 mins**

Ingredients

- ½ medium red onion, diced
- 8 oz. canned tuna
- 4 tbsp. mayonnaise
- 2 large eggs
- 2 oz. mozzarella cheese, shredded

Instructions

1. Cook the red onion in a well-oiled pan on medium heat for 5 minutes or until softened.
2. Drain the canned tuna and add it along with the rest of the ingredients to the pan. Salt and pepper everything to taste.
3. Stir the mixture together until the egg has cooked and the mozzarella has melted, about 2 minutes, and serve.

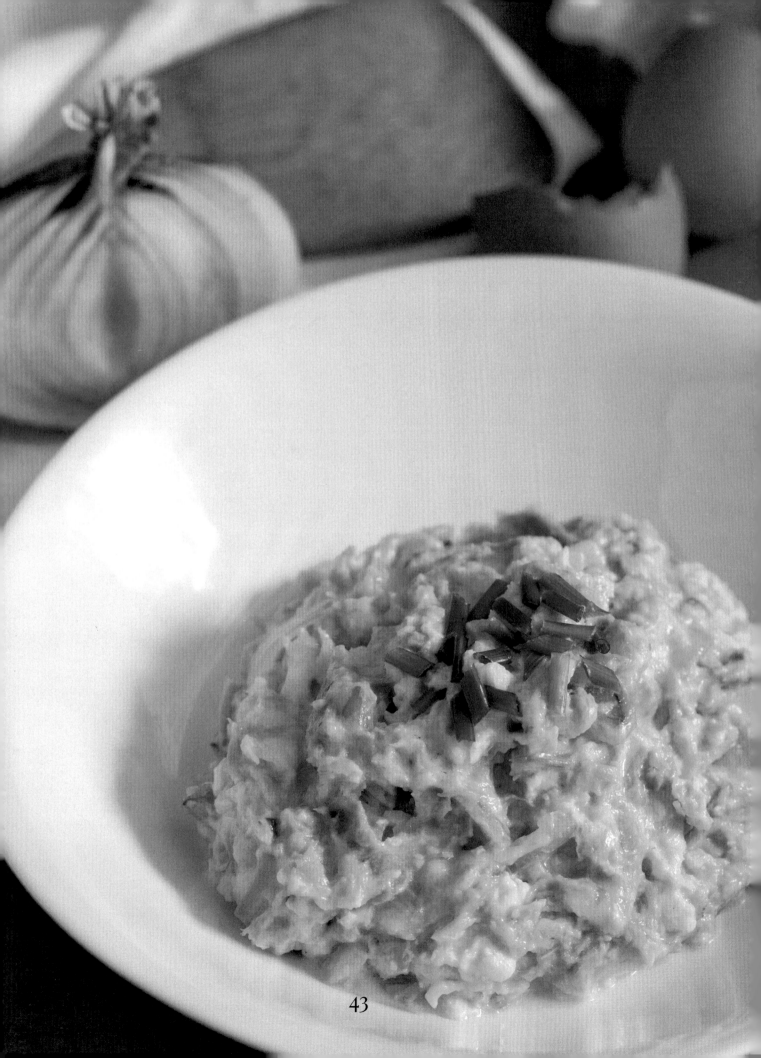

Roasted Tomato Soup

This creamy roasted tomato soup is naturally sweet and super velvety. It's perfect for cold winter mornings or even chilled on hot summer days!

Nutrition

330 calories per serving | Makes 4 servings

- 25 grams of fat
- 2 grams of protein
- 5 grams of net carbs

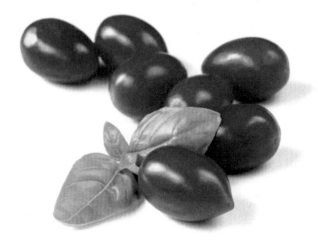

Ingredients

- 14 oz. plum tomatoes, halved
- 100 grams yellow onion, diced
- 4 tbsp. unsalted butter
- 1 cup heavy cream
- 1 bunch fresh basil

Instructions

1. Broil the tomatoes face down on a baking sheet in the oven until the skin is blistered, about 5–10 minutes. Rotate the pan occasionally to prevent burning. Let them cool slightly and peel and discard the skins.
2. In a lightly oiled soup pot on medium heat, cook the diced onion until translucent.
3. Add butter, cream, 2 cups of water and the roasted tomatoes. Season generously with salt and pepper.
4. Let the soup simmer for 20 minutes, adding the bunch of basil in the last 5 minutes.
5. Transfer everything to a blender and blend on high until smooth. Enjoy!

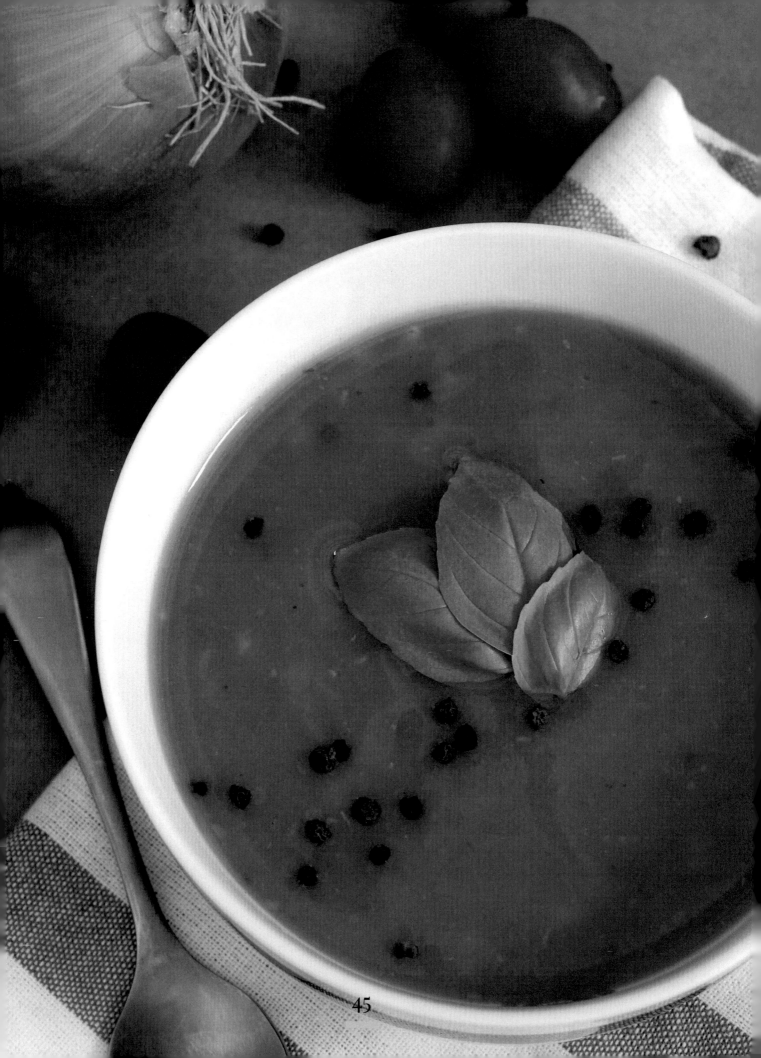

Poached Egg & Roasted Veg

Poached eggs are a favorite for brunch. Try this delicious, dairy-free option for lunch for a boost of healthy veggies and fats.

Nutrition

345 calories per serving | Makes 2 servings

- 25 grams of fat
- 20 grams of protein
- 5 grams of net carbs

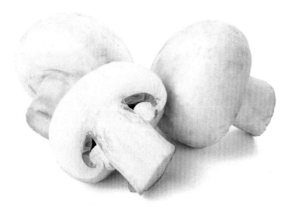

🕐 **Prep Time: 15 mins | Cook Time: 10 mins**

Ingredients

- 6 oz. white or brown mushrooms
- 10 spears asparagus
- 4 oz. breakfast sausage
- 1 roma tomato, chopped or sliced
- 2 large eggs, poached

Instructions

1. Chop the mushrooms and arrange them on a baking sheet with the asparagus. Drizzle with oil and broil for 4–6 minutes or until browned slightly.
2. Remove the sausage meat from its casing and cook it in a hot, oiled pan, breaking it up with a wooden spoon.
3. Combine the roasted veggies and fresh tomato on a plate and season with salt and pepper.
4. Add the cooked breakfast sausage and top with a poached egg. Enjoy!

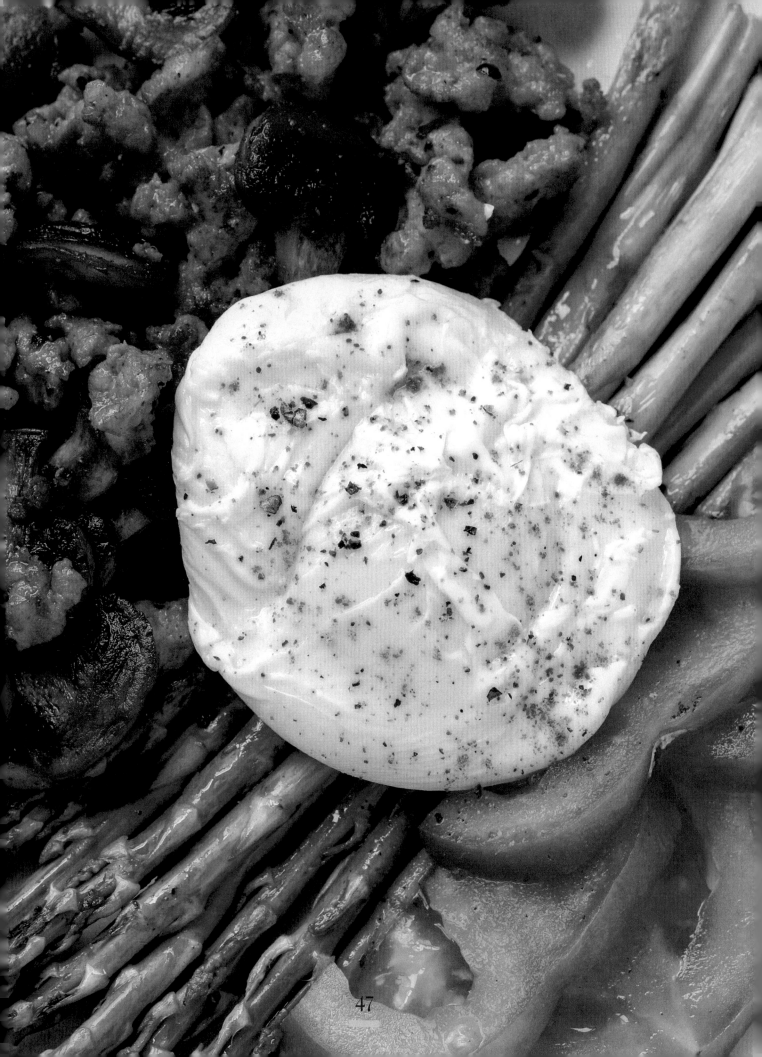

Traditional Egg Salad

It couldn't be simpler to make this creamy, tangy egg salad! Make a big batch and enjoy this tasty, low-carb lunch all week long.

Nutrition

350 calories per serving | Makes 2 servings

| 29 grams of fat
| 19 grams of protein
| 1 gram of net carbs

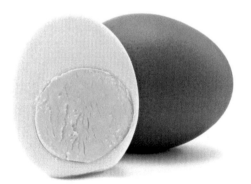

Ingredients

- 6 large eggs, boiled
- 3 tbsp. mayonnaise
- 2 tsp. fresh parsley, chopped
- 1 tsp. paprika
- 2 tsp. lemon juice

Instructions

1. Chop the boiled eggs and add them to a mixing bowl along with the rest of the ingredients.
2. Season everything with salt and pepper to taste and mix very well. The mixture should be more creamy than chunky, but it can vary based on preference.
3. Serve chilled and enjoy!

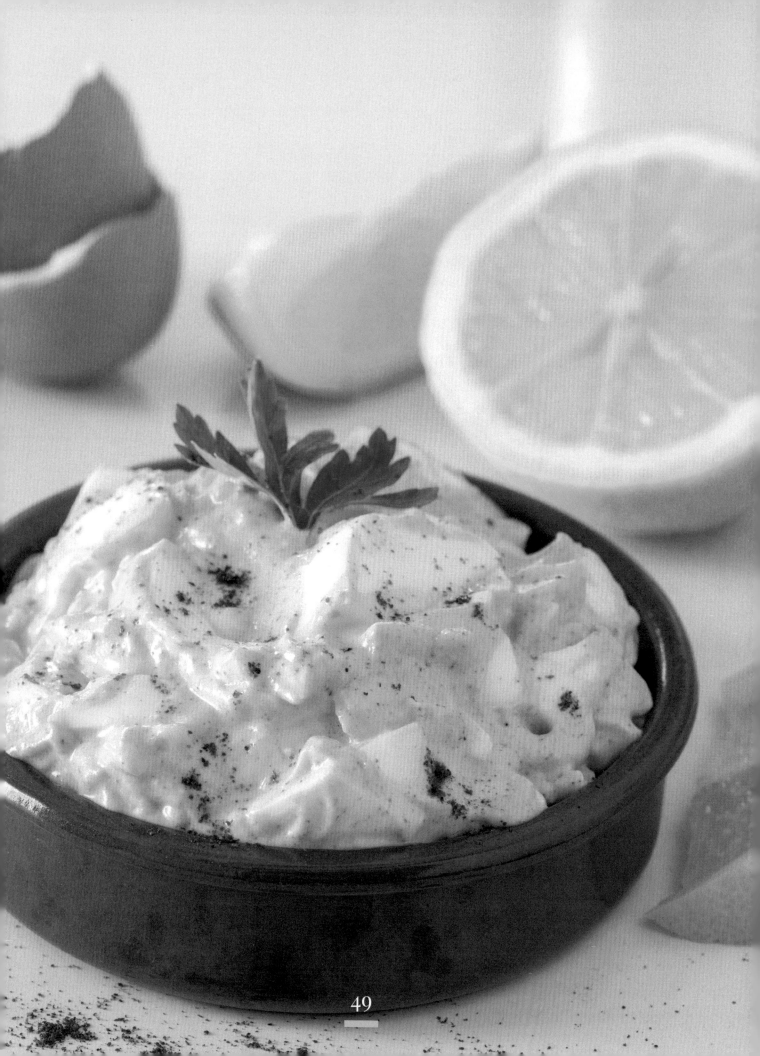

Bacon Cauliflower Chowder

The tasty flavor of bacon completes any soup! Try fried, crispy strips on a creamy cauliflower chowder for a light lunch.

Nutrition

275 calories per serving | Makes 4 servings

19 grams of fat

15 grams of protein

5 grams of net carbs

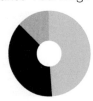

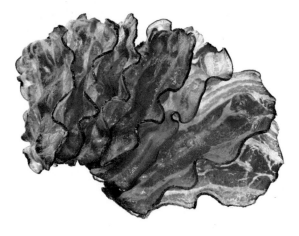

Ingredients

- 1 large cauliflower
- 1 white onion, diced
- 1 small carrot, shredded
- ½ cup sour cream
- 16 slices bacon

Instructions

1. Chop cauliflower and add the florets to an oiled soup pot with the onion and carrot. Season very well and cook until the onion is translucent and other vegetables are soft.
2. Add 4 cups of water and bring to a boil. Lower to a simmer for 1 hour, stirring occasionally.
3. In the last few minutes, mix in the sour cream.
4. Fry the bacon strips until crispy, chop them up and add to each soup bowl when serving.

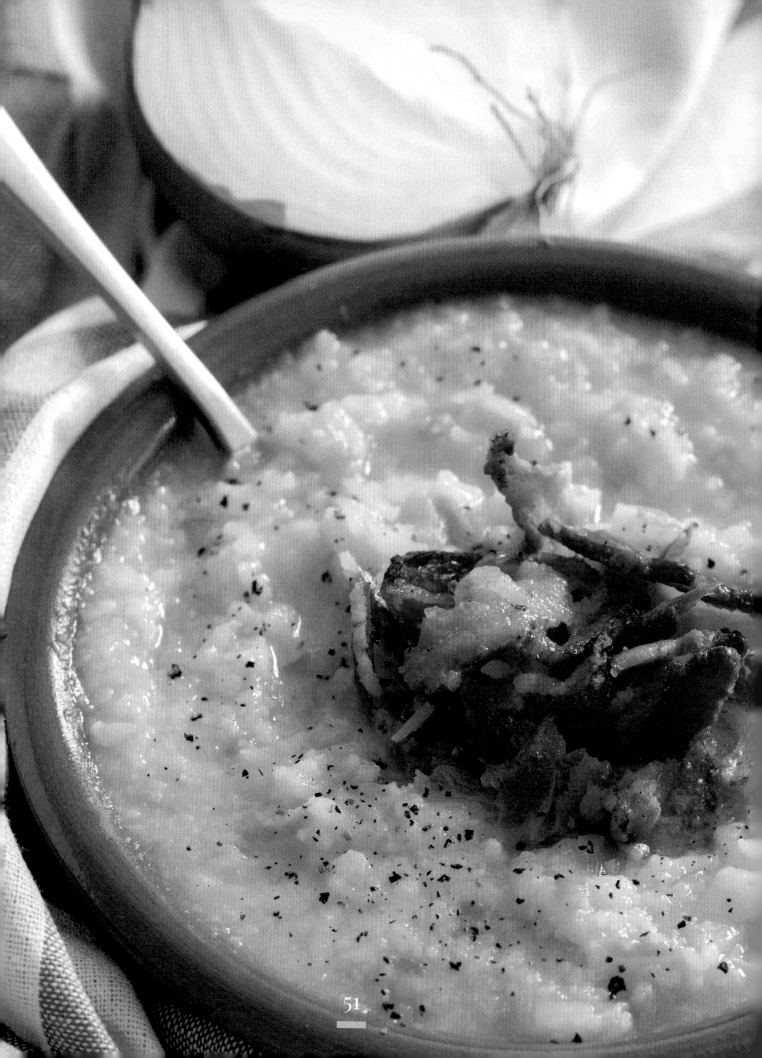

Chicken Avocado Salad

Grilled chicken and fresh avocado is lifted with the simple addition of lime juice! You'll swear this was a gourmet recipe!

Nutrition

300 calories per serving | Makes 2 servings

| 16 grams of fat
| 32 grams of protein
| 4 grams of net carbs

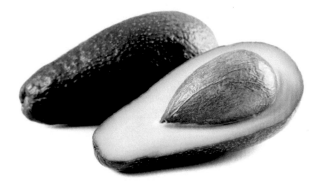

Ingredients

- 8 oz. boneless skinless chicken thighs
- 1 medium avocado
- 2 roma tomatoes
- 1 handful lettuce
- 1 lime, juiced

Instructions

1. Grill or fry the chicken thighs until fully cooked, about 5-8 minutes on each side.
2. Cube or slice the avocado and roma tomatoes. Shred the lettuce into bite-sized pieces.
3. Shred the chicken thighs using two forks or meat-shredding claws and combine everything in a large salad bowl.
4. Season with salt and pepper to taste and add the juice of a whole lime. Toss and enjoy!

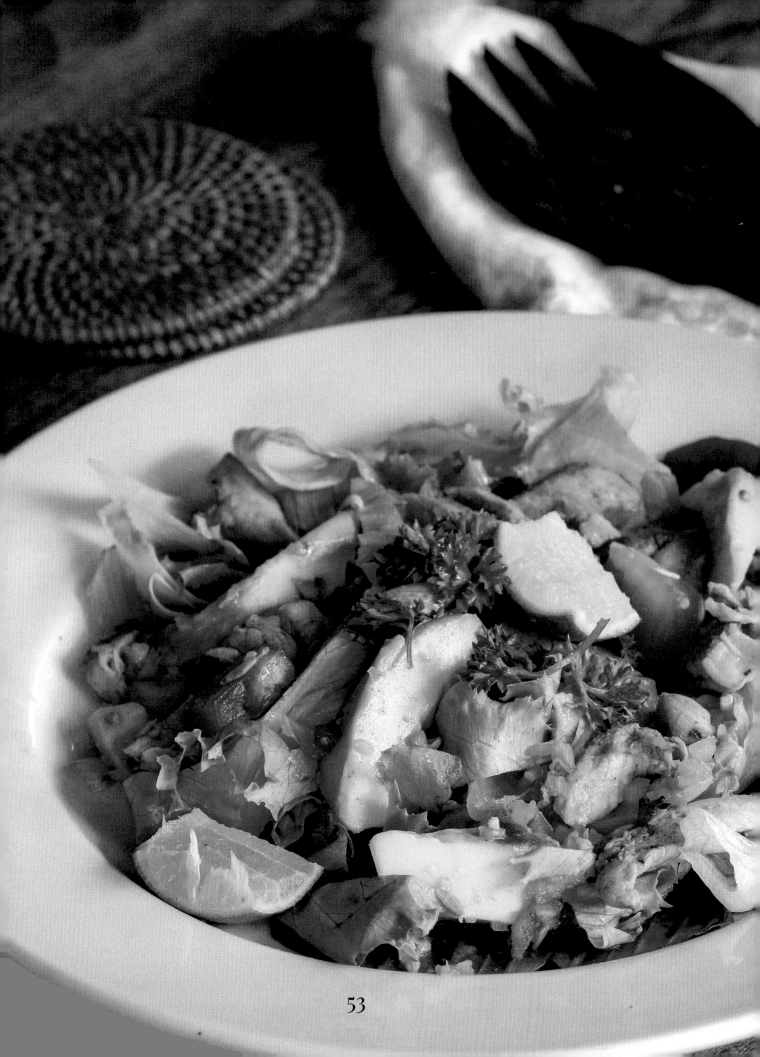

Juicy Tuna Salad

You can't beat the classics! We love this tuna salad recipe because it's juicy, packed with protein and fills you up fast!

Nutrition

375 calories per serving | Makes 2 servings

▮	22 grams of fat
▮	39 grams of protein
▮	4 grams of net carbs

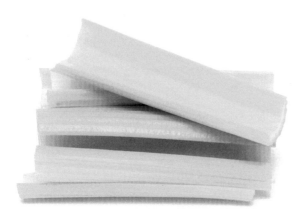

🕐 **Prep Time: 10 mins | Cook Time: 0 mins**

Ingredients

- 2 stalks celery
- ½ medium red onion
- 2 large eggs, boiled
- 12 oz. canned tuna
- 3 tbsp. mayonnaise

Instructions

1. Thinly chop the celery and dice the onion and eggs.
2. Drain the canned tuna and add all the ingredients into a bowl.
3. Salt and pepper to taste and mix everything well.
4. Serve and enjoy!

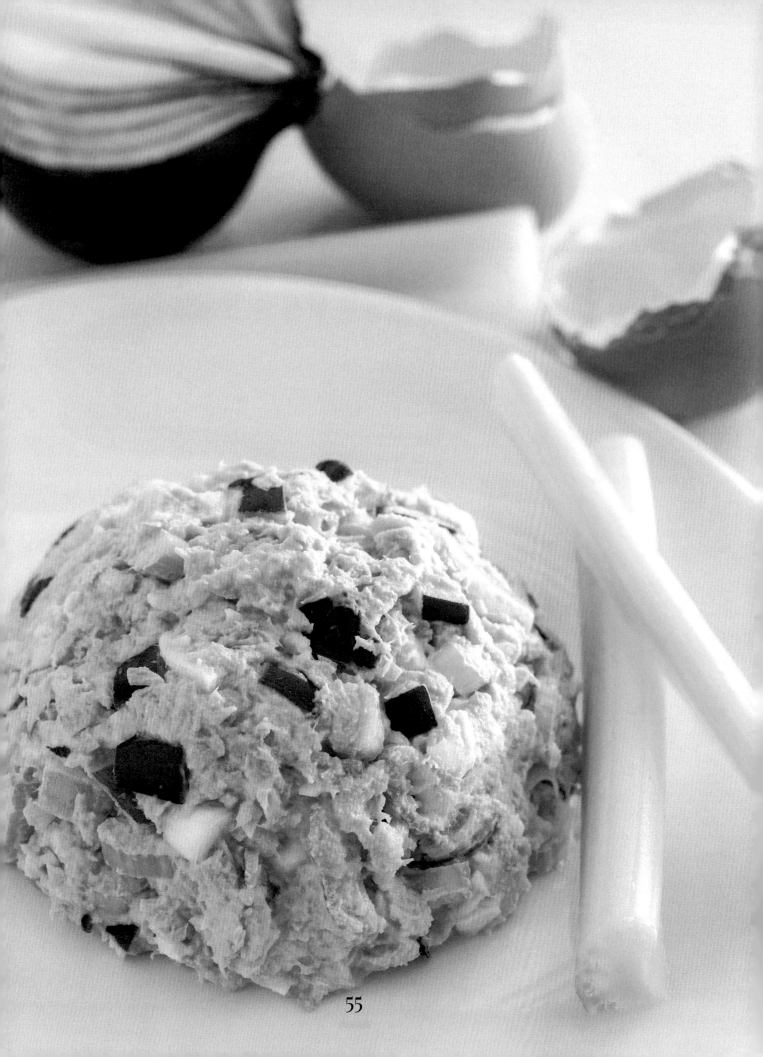

55

Coconut Macadamia Shake

Coconut cashew is one of the best flavor combos, but macadamias are much lower in carbs and higher in fat! So throw 'em in your lunch shake!

Nutrition

390 calories per serving | Makes 1 serving

- 38 grams of fat
- 3 grams of protein
- 4 grams of net carbs

🕐 **Prep Time: 5 mins | Cook Time: 0 mins**

Ingredients

- 2 cups unsweetened almond milk
- 1 oz. macadamia nuts
- ¼ cup unsweetened coconut flakes
- ½ tsp. ground cinnamon
- 10 drops liquid stevia

Instructions

1. Combine all the ingredients in a blender or Nutribullet and blend on high until very creamy, about 1–2 minutes.
2. Sweeten with stevia to taste. You can substitute with erythritol if you don't like the taste of stevia.
3. Serve cold and enjoy!

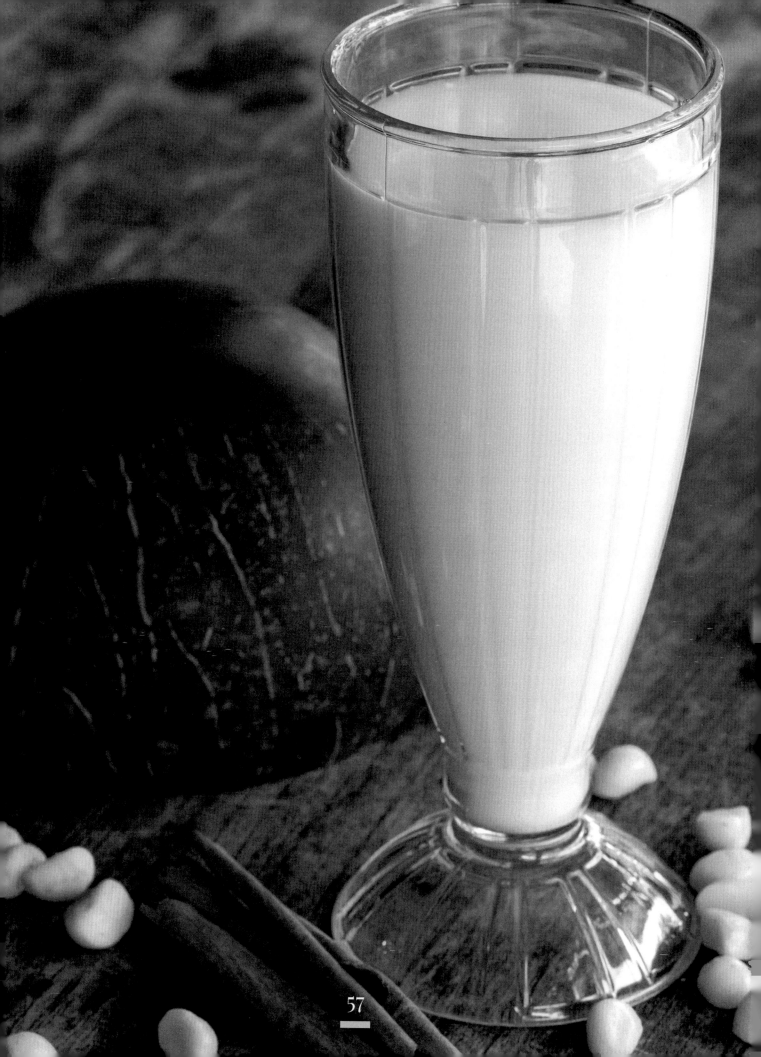

Cheddar Chips & Guacamole

This popular appetizer turned low-carb is surprisingly filling! Lots of healthy fats from avocado and cheddar cheese make this a delicious lunch.

Nutrition

420 calories per serving | Makes 1 serving

- 35 grams of fat
- 16 grams of protein
- 5 grams of net carbs

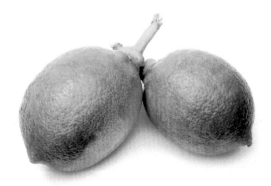

🕐 **Prep Time: 5 mins | Cook Time: 12 mins**

Ingredients

- 2 oz. cheddar cheese, shredded
- 1 avocado
- ½ roma tomato, diced
- 1 tbsp. white onion, diced
- 1 tbsp. lime juice

Instructions

1. Add the shredded cheddar in a thin layer to a pan on medium heat. Let it melt and caramelize until golden all around, about 10 minutes. When it has solidified and browned a bit, flip it and cook for another 2 minutes.
2. Mash together the avocado, tomato, onion and lime juice. Season with salt and pepper.
3. Serve together and enjoy!

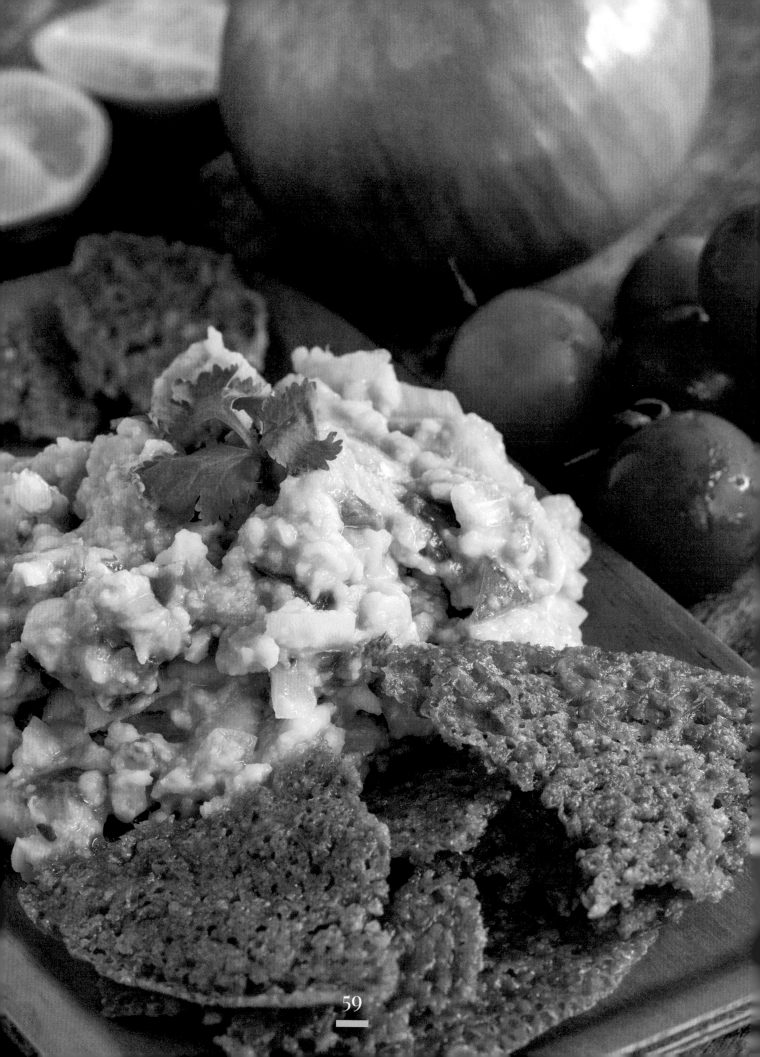

Chicken Salad-Stuffed Avocado

Avocado shells are a great alternative to boring bowls! We love adding in creamy chicken salad and being the envy of our friends.

Nutrition

570 calories per serving | Makes 1 serving

- 45 grams of fat
- 29 grams of protein
- 5 grams of net carbs

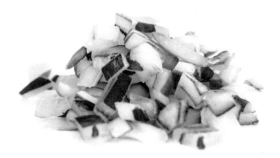

🕐 **Prep Time: 10 mins | Cook Time: 10 mins**

Ingredients

- 3 oz. chicken breast
- 1 tbsp. red onion, diced
- 1 celery stalk, diced
- 1 medium avocado
- ⅓ cup sour cream

Instructions

1. Cook the chicken on low heat until fully cooked. Then shred it using two forks.
2. Combine chicken, onion and celery in a bowl.
3. Cut and pit an avocado. Scoop some of the avocado out and add it to the bowl.
4. Add in the sour cream, salt and pepper to the bowl and toss everything well.
5. Scoop the chicken salad mix back into the avocado halves and enjoy!

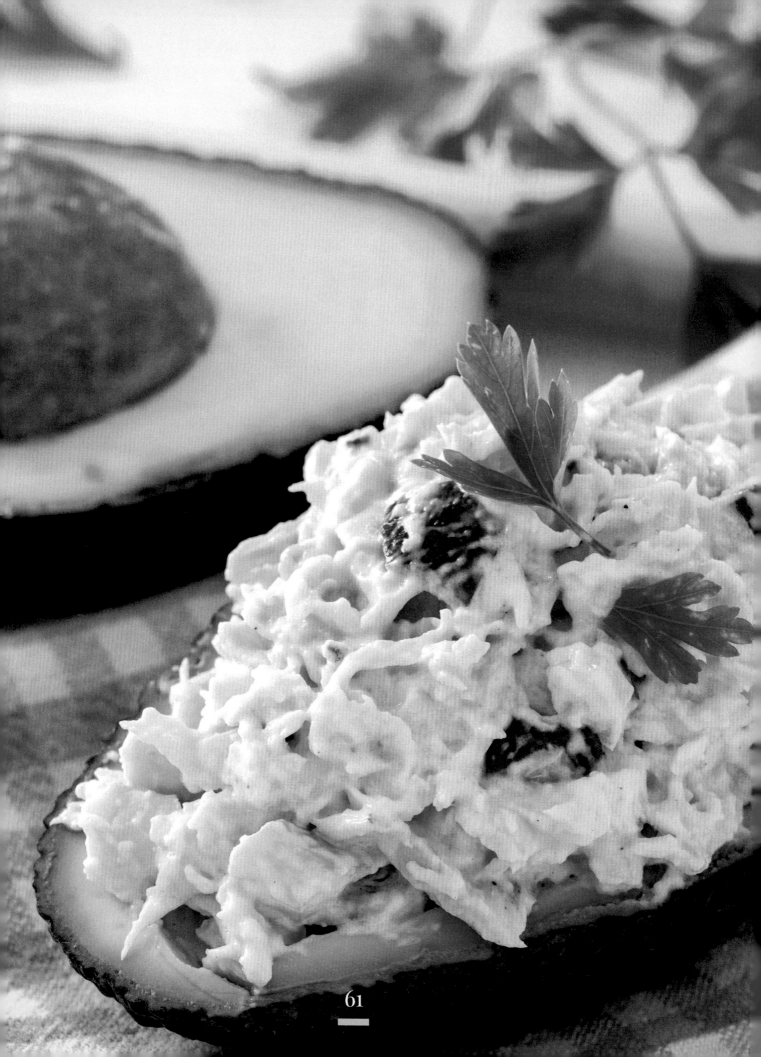

Cashew Chicken Stir-Fry

Here's a lighter lunch option that you can always add to! Asian veggies and *Miracle Rice* makes this a great alternative to unhealthy take-out.

Nutrition

285 calories per serving | Makes 4 servings

- 17 grams of fat
- 28 grams of protein
- 4.5 grams of net carbs

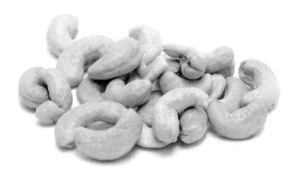

Ingredients

- 2 bags *Miracle Noodle* Rice
- 1 lb. boneless skinless chicken thighs, cubed
- 20 spears asparagus
- ½ cup whole cashews
- 2 tbsp. soy sauce

Instructions

1. Prepare the *Miracle Noodle Rice* according to the package instructions.
2. Cook the chicken thighs in a well-oiled pan on medium heat until almost fully cooked.
3. Cut the fibrous ends off the asparagus (about 2 inches). Add the asparagus, cashews and soy sauce into the pan.
4. Let simmer, stirring, for 8 minutes.
5. Add *Miracle Rice*, stir for 2 minutes and serve.

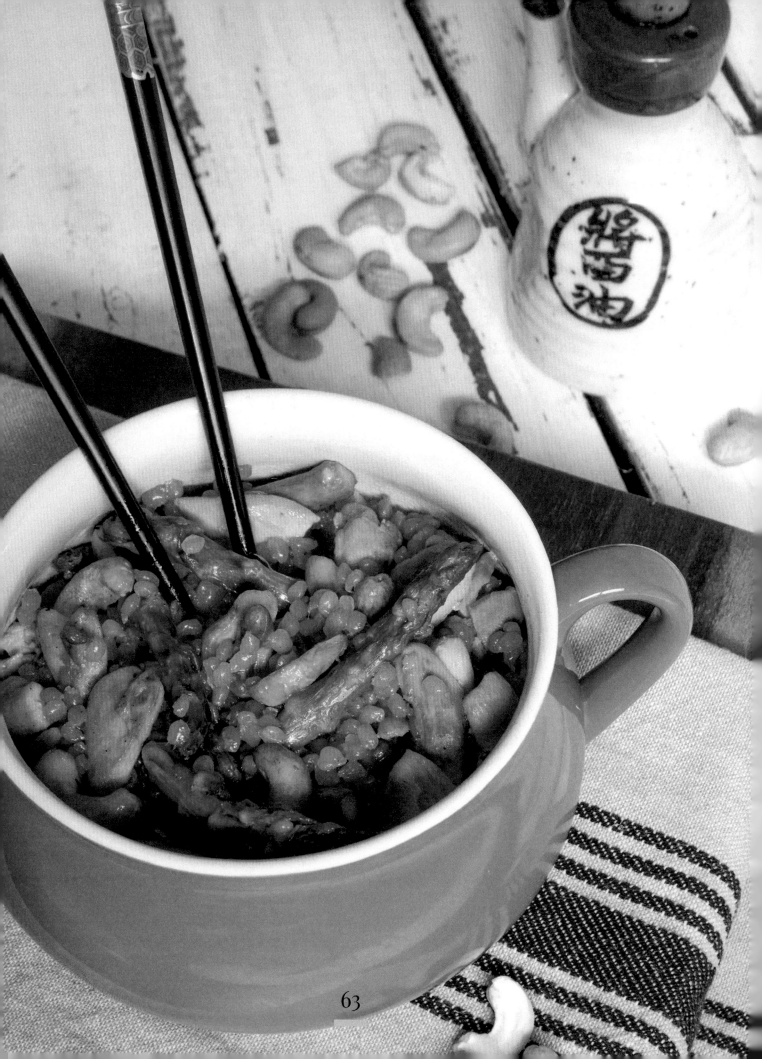

Chicken-Wrapped Bacon Bites

Finger foods make eating fun! Be the envy of your coworkers when you whip these out of your lunchbox at break time!

Nutrition

575 calories per serving | Makes 2 servings

▌ 44 grams of fat

▌ 44 grams of protein

▌ 2 grams of net carbs

🕐 **Prep Time: 15 mins | Cook Time: 10 mins**

Ingredients

- 6 strips bacon
- 4 oz. chicken breast
- 2 stalks green onion
- 2 tbsp. mayonnaise
- 1 tsp. hot sauce of choice

Instructions

1. Cut the bacon in half to make 12 strips.
2. Cube the chicken into 12 bite-sized pieces and chop the green onion into 2″ pieces.
3. Place a chicken cube and green onion piece onto the end of one bacon strip and roll the bacon tightly wrapping the contents.
4. Cook on a lightly oiled pan on medium heat for about 10 minutes, flipping occasionally.
5. Serve with mayonnaise mixed with hot sauce.

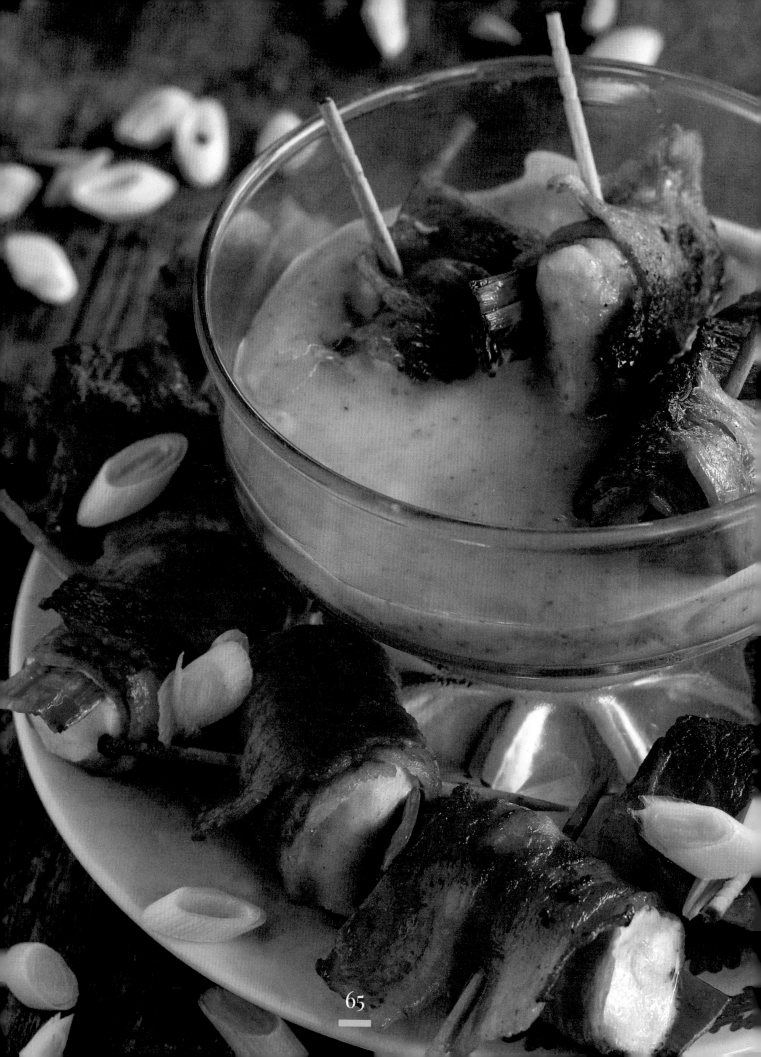

Lemon Kale Salad

You can keep this lemon kale salad vegetarian, or add your favorite protein to it. It's fresh, tangy and so easy to make.

Nutrition

420 calories per serving | Makes 2 servings

41 grams of fat

9 grams of protein

5 grams of net carbs

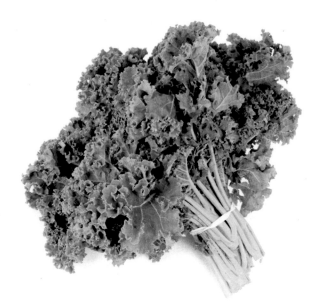

Ingredients

- 4 oz. fresh kale
- 2 oz. feta cheese
- 30 grams slivered almonds
- 1 lemon, juiced
- ¼ cup olive oil

Instructions

1. Rinse and rip the kale leaves and add them to a salad bowl with the lemon juice and olive oil. Massage for a few minutes to soften the leaves.
2. Crumble the feta into the bowl and add the slivered almonds.
3. Season with a bit of salt, toss well and enjoy!

Tip: Massaging the kale leaves with lemon juice and olive oil will help them soften and become less bitter.

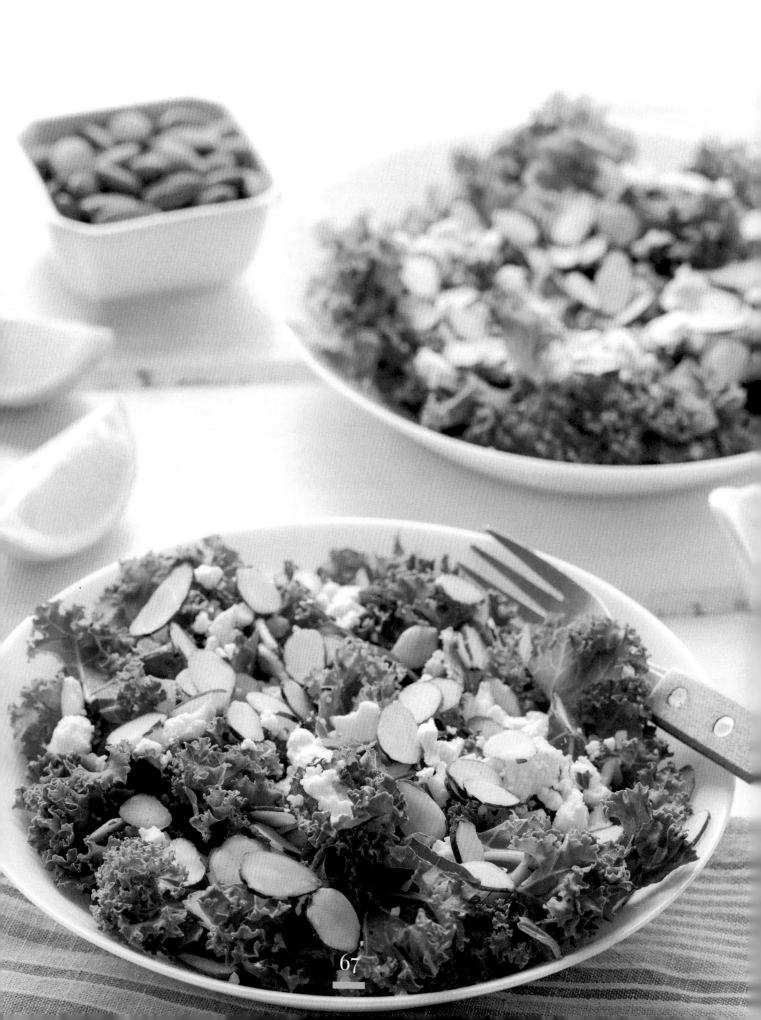

Cheeseburger Crepes

You'll wonder why you didn't think of this sooner — cheeseburger stuffed savory crepes! Super low-carb and super portable!

Nutrition

520 calories per serving | Makes 2 servings

- 36 grams of fat
- 38 grams of protein
- 3.5 grams of net carbs

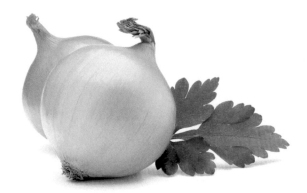

Ingredients

- ½ yellow onion, diced
- ½ lb. ground beef
- 2 oz. cheddar cheese
- 2 large eggs
- 2 oz. cream cheese

Instructions

1. Fry the onion and ground beef in an oiled pan on medium heat for 5 minutes. Add cheddar and mix well until melted.
2. Whisk the eggs and cream cheese together in a bowl until smooth. Add ¼ of the batter to a very hot, oiled pan. Tilt to coat the pan evenly and fry for 2 minutes. Flip and fry for 2 another minutes. Repeat for the rest of the batter.
3. Add the beef cheeseburger mix to the crepes and roll them up.
4. Slice in half and serve 2 full crepes (4 halves) per serving.

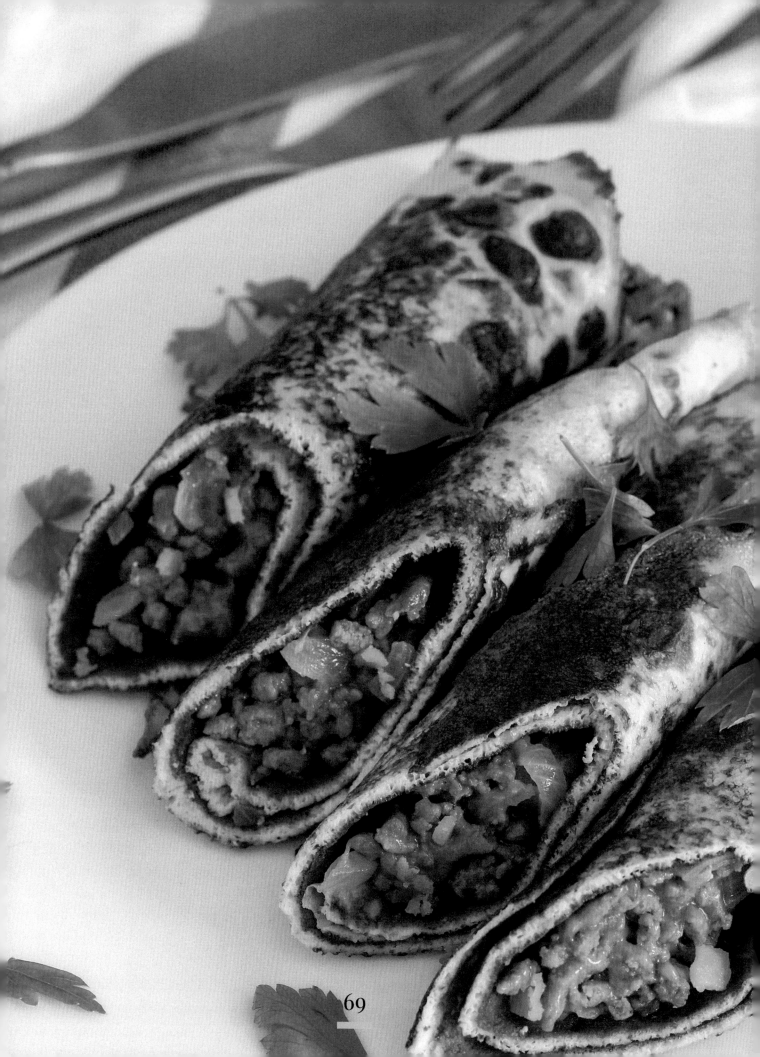

Pizza Casserole

This delicious pizza casserole includes the best part of any pizza but without the crust and a few extra tasty ingredients!

Nutrition

500 calories per serving | Makes 4 servings

- 34 grams of fat
- 42 grams of protein
- 5 grams of net carbs

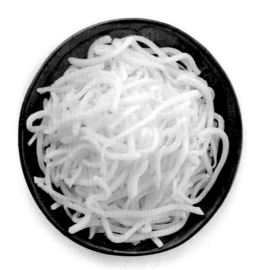

🕐 **Prep Time: 15 mins | Cook Time: 35 mins**

Ingredients

- 1 lb. boneless skinless chicken thighs
- 12 oz. ricotta cheese
- 2 large zucchini, cubed
- 4 oz. pepperoni, sliced
- 1 cup shredded mozzarella (see p. 26)

Instructions

1. Fry the chicken thighs in an oiled pan on medium heat until cooked. Shred with 2 forks or meat-shredding claws.
2. Combine the ricotta, chicken, zucchini, half of the pepperoni slices, salt and pepper in a 9×13" casserole dish and bake for 25 minutes at 350°F.
3. In last 5 minutes of baking, top with shredded mozzarella and the rest of the pepperoni slices. Finish baking and serve!

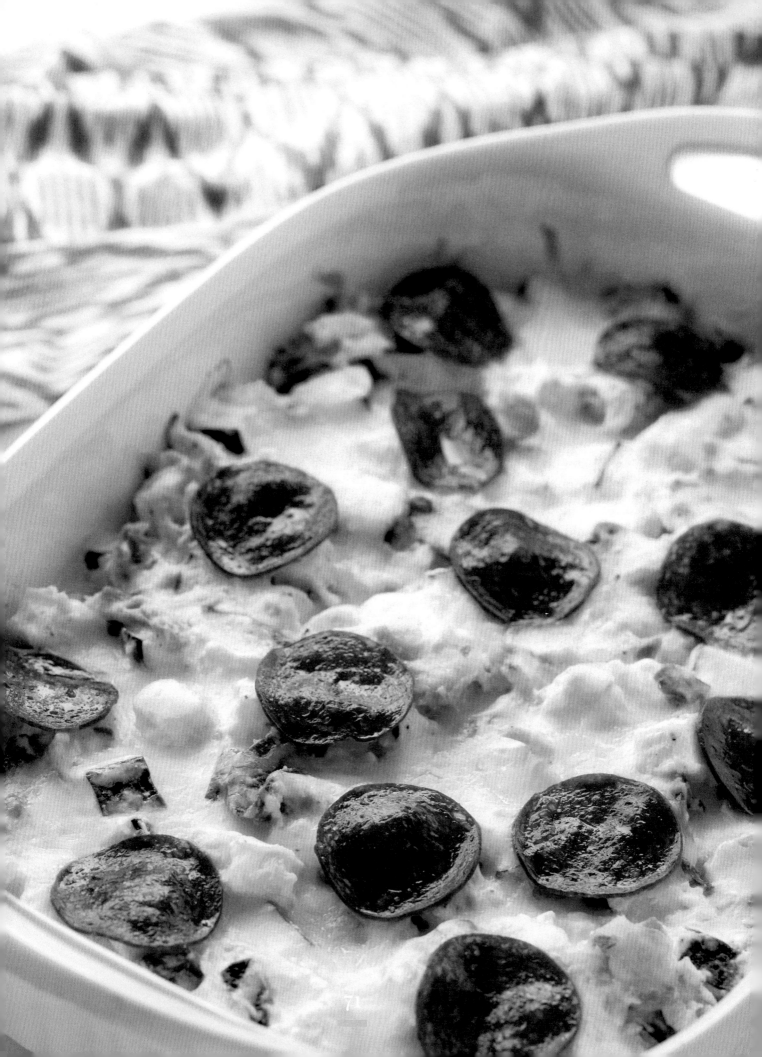

Taco Salad Bowl

You'll forget all about taco shells when you dig in to this taco salad bowl. It's got all the yummy flavors of a taco without all the carbs!

Nutrition

465 calories per serving | Makes 2 servings

- 33 grams of fat
- 31 grams of protein
- 4 grams of net carbs

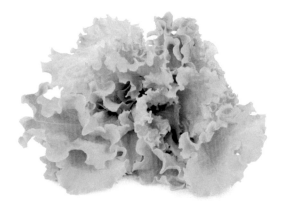

Ingredients

- ½ lb. ground beef
- 1 small avocado
- 2 roma tomatoes
- 1 handful lettuce
- ½ cup shredded cheddar

Instructions

1. Brown the ground beef in a hot, oiled pan.
2. While it's cooking, cube the avocado and roma tomatoes.
3. Shred the lettuce into a salad bowl and add the avocado and roma tomatoes.
4. Throw in the ground beef and cheddar. Salt and pepper to taste.
5. Mix to combine everything and serve.

Tip: *For a quick dressing, just use a dollop of sour cream!*

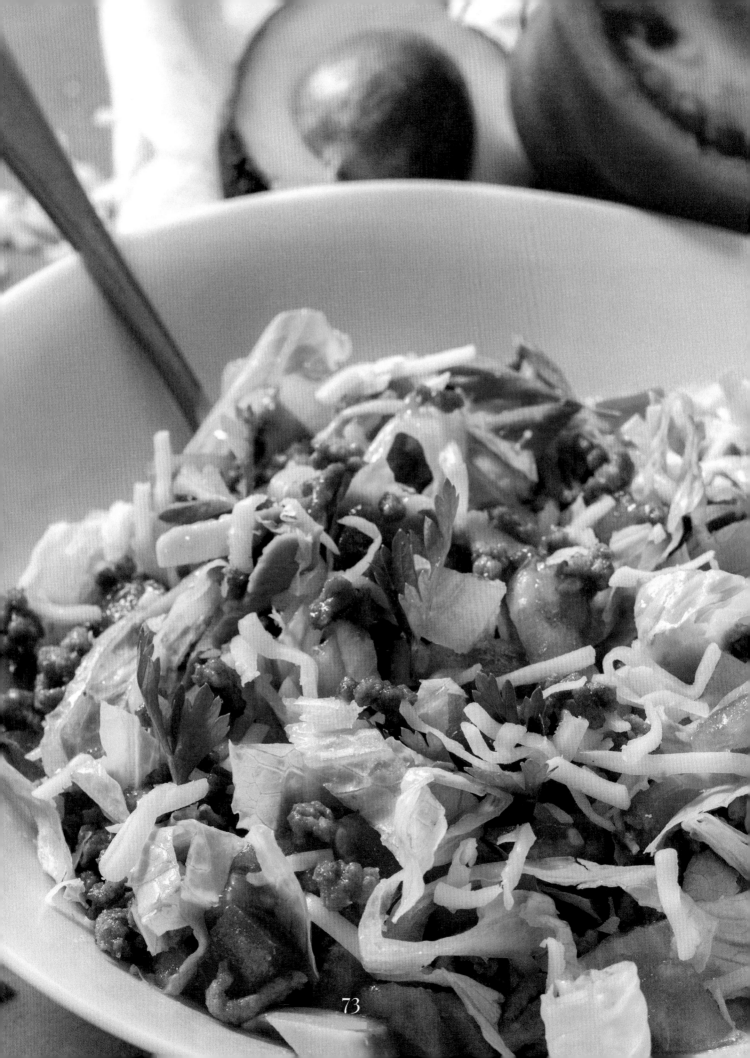

Meatball Marinara Bake

Who needs spaghetti when you can make delicious, moist meatballs and enjoy them with loads of cheese? Best of all, you only need one pan!

Nutrition

420 calories per serving | Makes 8 servings

- 29 grams of fat
- 38 grams of protein
- 3 grams of net carbs

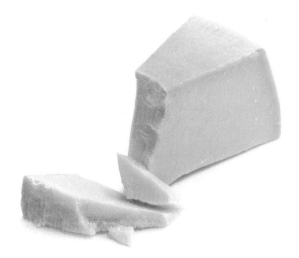

Ingredients

- 1 ½ lbs. ground beef
- 4 large eggs
- 1 cup grated Parmesan cheese
- 2 cups marinara sauce
- 2 cups shredded mozzarella

Instructions

1. Combine the beef, eggs, Parmesan and ½ teaspoon of salt. Make 1–1.5" inch meatballs.
2. In an oiled pan on high heat, sear the meatballs on all sides for about 3–5 minutes until they're browned.
3. Into a 9×9" casserole dish, add the marinara sauce and meatballs and bake for 20 minutes at 350°F.
4. Add mozzarella, broil for 2 minutes and serve.

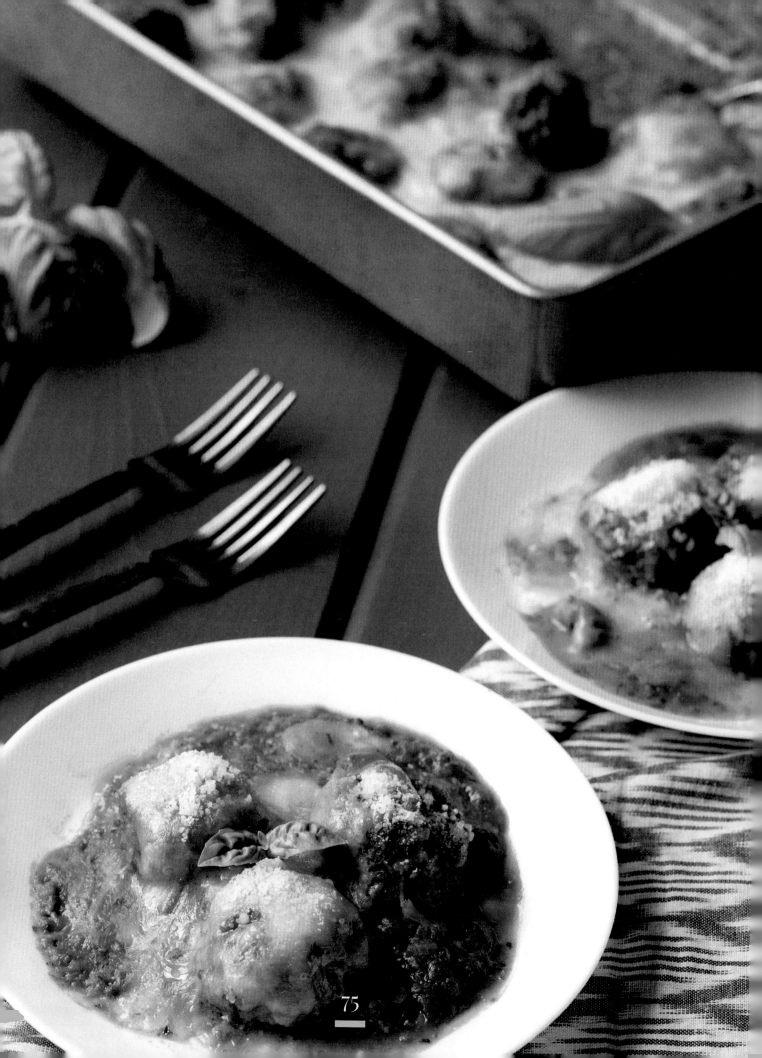

Creamy Shrimp Curry

Shrimp often goes unnoticed in a sea of meat-laden dishes, but their texture really stands out in our delicate, creamy curry.

Nutrition

329 calories per serving | Makes 2 servings

- 18 grams of fat
- 49 grams of protein
- 5 grams of net carbs

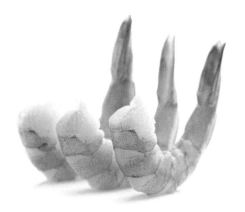

🕒 **Prep Time: 5 mins | Cook Time: 10 mins**

Ingredients

- 1 large zucchini, diced
- 12 oz. large shrimp, peeled
- 2 tbsp. shelled edamame
- 1 tbsp. soy sauce
- 4 oz. cream cheese

Instructions

1. In an oiled pan on medium heat, fry the diced zucchini for about 7 minutes, stirring often.
2. Add the shrimp and let cook until fully pink.
3. Add in edamame, soy sauce and cream cheese to the pan and stir well for an additional 2 minutes or until the cream cheese has melted.
4. Salt and pepper to taste, serve and enjoy!

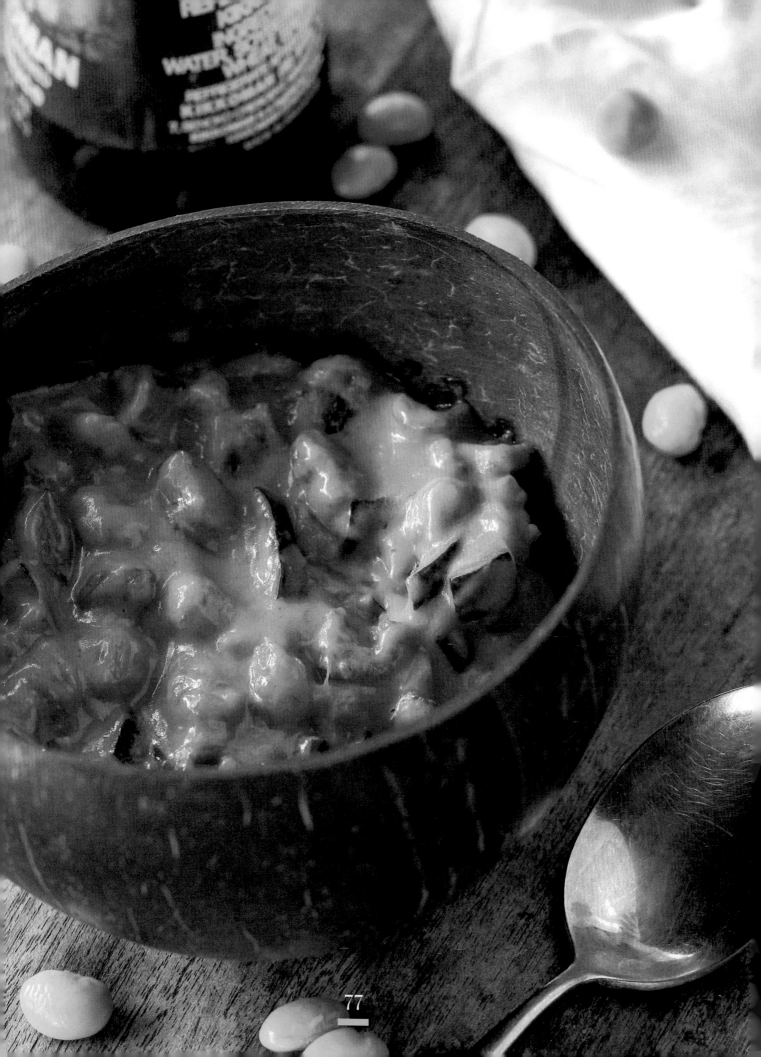

Loaded Cobb Salad

Cobb salads are a safe, low-carb option in restaurants, but who needs a restaurant to enjoy it? Make your own super filling lunch and enjoy!

Nutrition

400 calories per serving | Makes 2 servings

■ 36 grams of fat

■ 13 grams of protein

■ 3 grams of net carbs

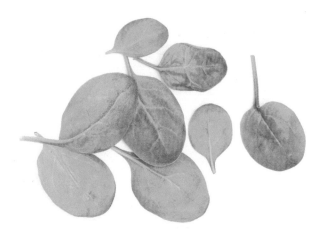

🕐 **Prep Time: 10 mins | Cook Time: 5 mins**

Ingredients

- 4 strips bacon, chopped
- 2 handfuls baby spinach
- 2 large eggs, hard boiled
- 1 small avocado
- 3 tbsp. ranch dressing

Instructions

1. Fry the chopped bacon in a pan on medium heat until you have crispy bite-sized pieces.
2. In the meantime, make a bed of baby spinach in two bowls.
3. Chop the eggs and avocado and divide them evenly into each bowl on top of the bed of baby spinach.
4. Add the fried bacon bits to each salad.
5. Top each salad with ranch dressing and serve!

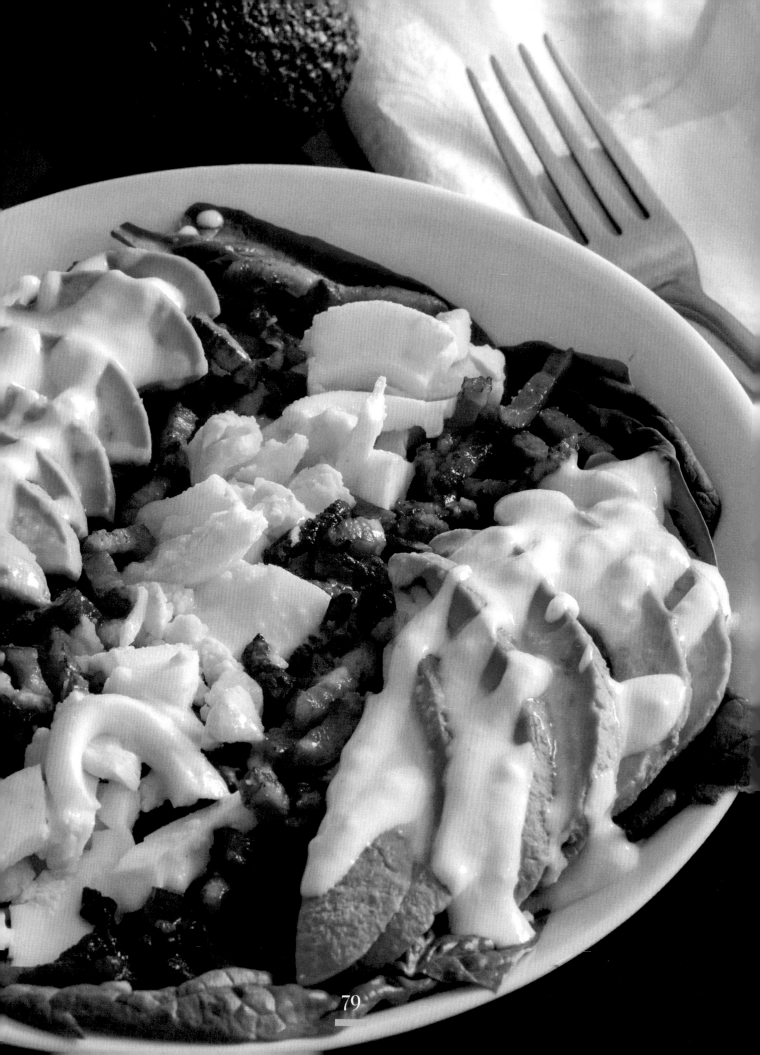

Creamy Peppercorn Beef

Juicy beef only gets juicier with the addition of cream and the sweetness of onion. Try it on a bed of lettuce for some added crunch!

Nutrition

630 calories per serving | Makes 2 servings

- 50 grams of fat
- 46 grams of protein
- 4.5 grams of net carbs

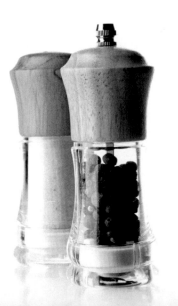

🕐 **Prep Time: 10 mins | Cook Time: 30 mins**

Ingredients

- ½ white onion, sliced
- 1 lb. sirloin steak
- ¾ cup heavy cream
- 2 tbsp. peppercorns
- 2 handfuls romaine lettuce

Instructions

1. In an oiled pan on medium heat, cook onions until translucent, then take them off the pan.
2. Turn the heat up to high and when the pan is very hot, sear the sirloin steak for 5 minutes on each side. Then, slice the steak into strips.
3. Place onion and steak strips back into the pan with the cream and peppercorns. Salt to taste. Simmer for 5–10 mins and serve over a bed of romaine lettuce.

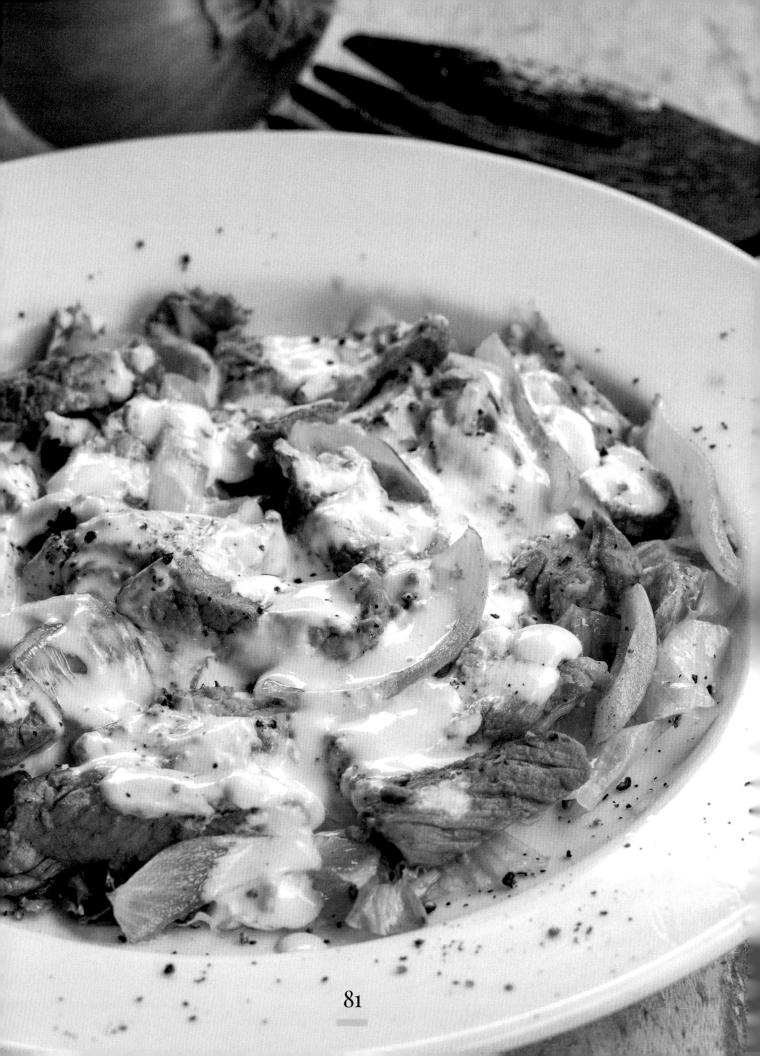

Bacon Turkey Wraps

Nothing beats some refreshing lettuce wraps. Forgo the processed, low-carb wraps in favor of something all natural!

Nutrition

585 calories per serving | Makes 1 serving

44 grams of fat

43 grams of protein

2 grams of net carbs

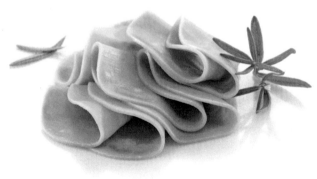

Ingredients

- 3 strips bacon
- 3 tsp. mayonnaise
- 3 lettuce leaves
- 3 oz. provolone cheese
- 3 oz. sliced turkey

Instructions

1. Cook bacon until crispy, then chop it into bits.
2. Add a teaspoon of mayonnaise to each lettuce leaf and then top each with a slice of provolone cheese.
3. Lay a slice of turkey onto each wrap and then sprinkle with the cooked bacon.
4. Roll each up tightly and enjoy or pack away!

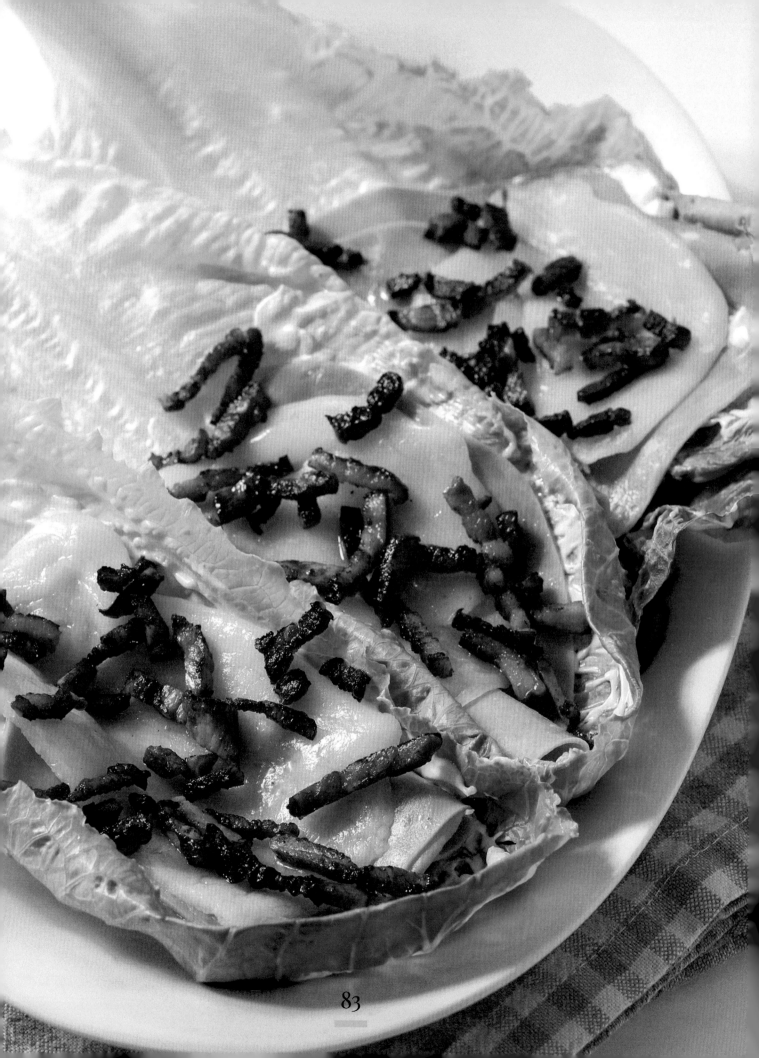

Creamy Mushroom Soup

Delicate and creamy — this soup is quick to make and tastes like it's straight out of a restaurant! You'd never guess it's only got 5 ingredients.

Nutrition

320 calories per serving | Makes 4 servings

- 23 grams of fat
- 28 grams of protein
- 5 grams of net carbs

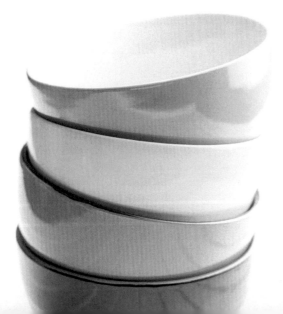

🕐 **Prep Time: 15 mins | Cook Time: 50 mins**

Ingredients

- 4 cups chicken broth
- ½ medium yellow onion, diced
- 12 oz. white or brown mushrooms, chopped
- 1 lb. boneless skinless chicken thighs
- ¾ cup heavy cream

Instructions

1. Add chicken broth, onion and mushrooms to a soup pot on medium heat.
2. Once at a boil, reduce heat to a simmer for 30 minutes. Salt and pepper to taste.
3. Fry chicken in an oiled pan on medium heat until cooked, about 6 minutes, then shred.
4. Add the chicken thighs and heavy cream to the pot and cook for an additional 10 minutes. Serve and enjoy!

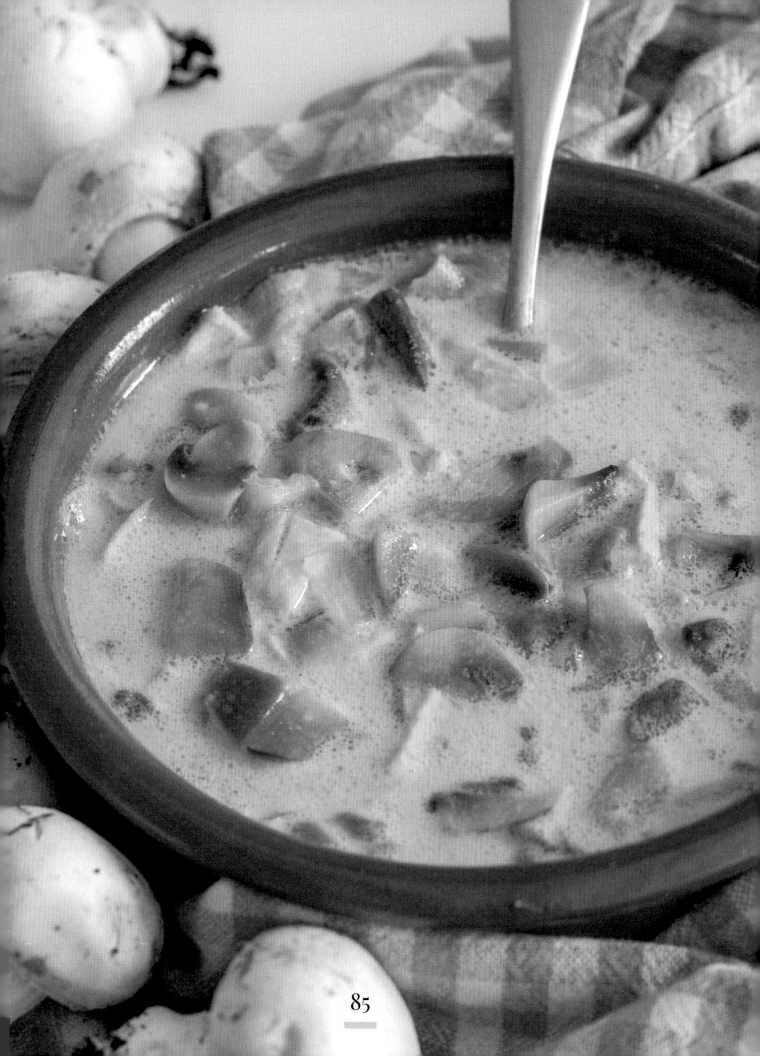

Cabbage & Sausage Skillet

You'd never think two things like sausage and cabbage could go together so perfectly! Wilted cabbage is very reminiscent of noodles.

Nutrition

310 calories per serving | Makes 4 servings

■ 25 grams of fat

■ 13 grams of protein

■ 5 grams of net carbs

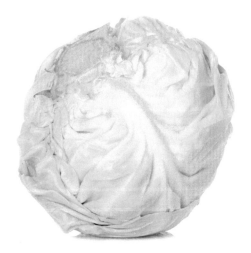

Ingredients

- 4 Italian sausage links
- ½ head green cabbage, shredded
- 2 tbsp. unsalted butter
- ¼ cup sour cream
- ¼ cup mayonnaise

Instructions

1. Fully cook the sausage links in a pan and then slice them into bite-sized pieces.
2. In the same pan, wilt the cabbage in the butter, stirring occasionally.
3. Add the sausages back into the pan and add the sour cream and mayonnaise.
4. Season with salt and pepper and let simmer for about 10 minutes, stirring occasionally.

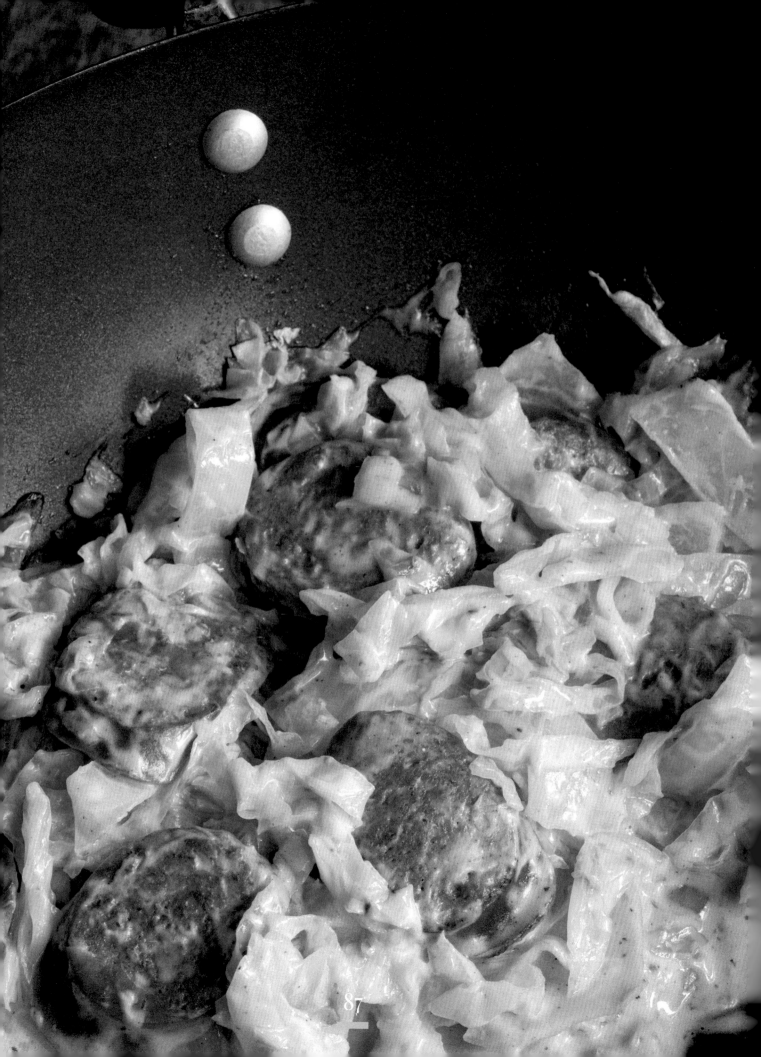

Thank You

Our hopes are that some of these lunches will become staples in your diet making low-carb cooking more delicious and easier for you on a daily basis.

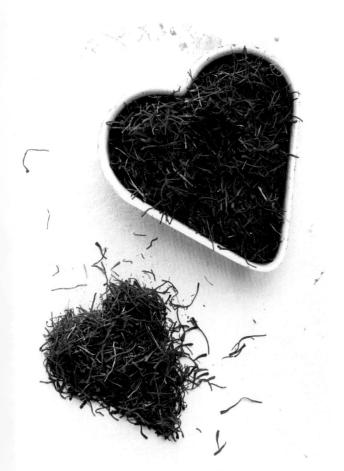

If you have questions, suggestions or any other feedback, please don't hesitate to contact us directly: hello@tasteaholics.com.

We answer emails every day and we'd love to hear from you. Each comment we receive is valuable and helps us in continuing to provide quality content.

Your direct feedback could be used to help others discover the benefits of going low-carb!

If you have a success story, please send it to us! We're always happy to hear about our readers' success.

Thank you again and we hope you have enjoyed *Lunch in Five*!

— *Vicky Ushakova & Rami Abramov*

About the Authors

Vicky Ushakova and Rami Abramov co-founded Tasteaholics.com to provide an easy way to understand why the ketogenic diet is truly effective for weight loss and health management. They create recipes that are low-carb, high-fat and maximize flavor. The books in their *Keto in Five* series are wildly popular among the low-carb community due to their simplicity and efficacy.

Vicky and Rami's mission is to continue to improve their audience's health and outlook on life through diet and nutrition education. They are dedicated to helping change the detrimental nutritional guidelines in the United States and across the globe that have been plaguing millions of people over the last 40 years.

The duo travels the world to explore new cultures, cuisines and culinary techniques which they pass on through new recipes and content available on their website.

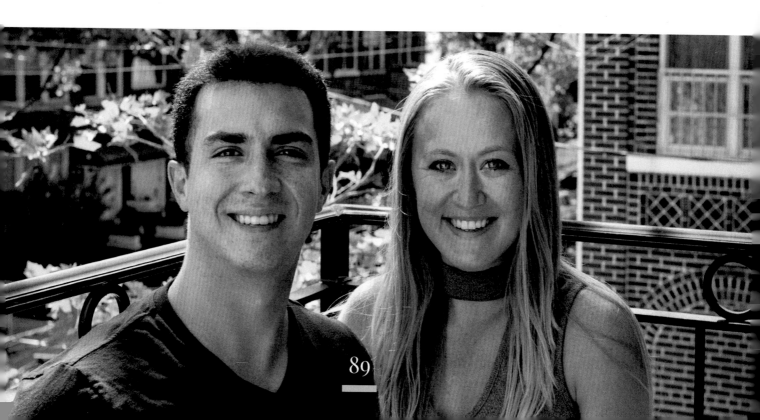

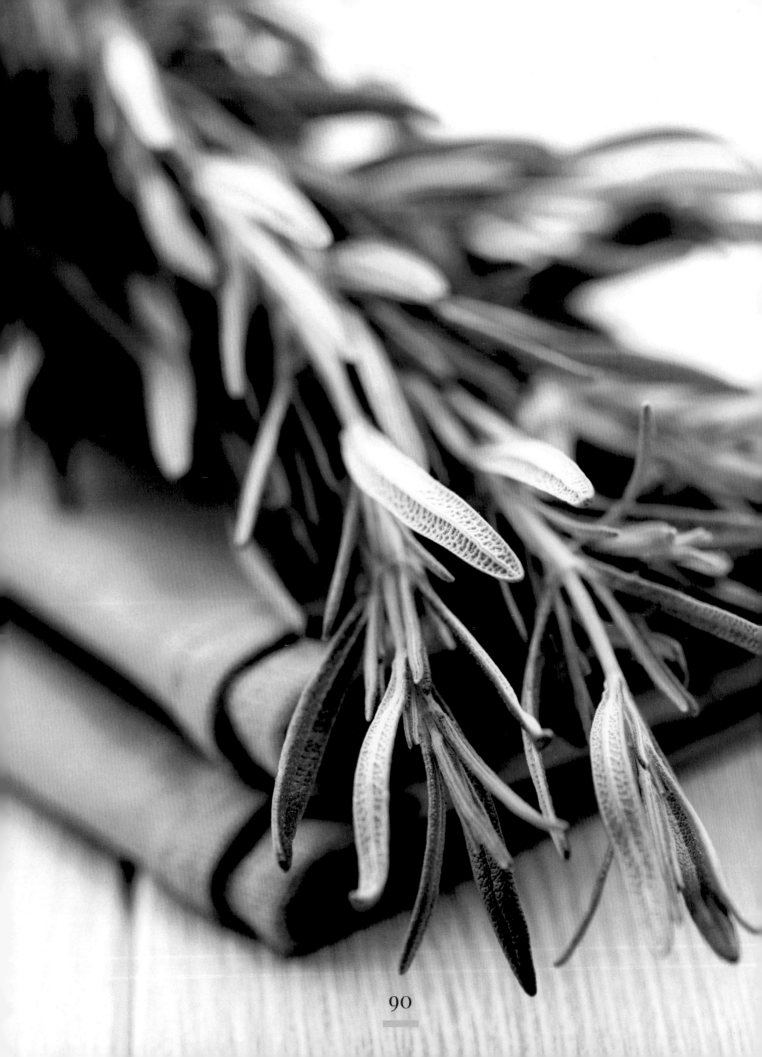

Personal Notes

Use these pages to write down any recipe notes and more delicious ideas.

References

1. Aude, Y., A. S, Agatston, F. Lopez-Jimenez, et al. "The National Cholesterol Education Program Diet vs a Diet Lower in Carbohydrates and Higher in Protein and Monounsaturated Fat: A Randomized Trial." JAMA Internal Medicine 164, no. 19 (2004): 2141–46. doi: 10.1001/archinte.164.19.2141. jamanetwork.com/journals/jamainternalmedicine/article-abstract/217514.

2. De Lau, L. M., M. Bornebroek, J. C. Witteman, A. Hofman, P. J. Koudstaal, and M. M. Breteler. "Dietary Fatty Acids and the Risk of Parkinson Disease: The Rotterdam Study." Neurology 64, no. 12 (June 2005): 2040–5. doi:10.1212/01.WNL.0000166038.67153.9F. www.ncbi.nlm.nih.gov/pubmed/15985568/.

3. Freeman, J. M., E. P. Vining, D. J. Pillas, P. L. Pyzik, J. C. Casey, and L M. Kelly. "The Efficacy of the Ketogenic Diet-1998: A Prospective Evaluation of Intervention in 150 Children." Pediatrics 102, no. 6 (December 1998): 1358–63. www.ncbi.nlm.nih.gov/pubmed/9832569/.

4. Hemingway, C, J. M. Freeman, D. J. Pillas, and P. L. Pyzik. "The Ketogenic Diet: A 3- to 6-Year Follow-up of 150 Children Enrolled Prospectively. Pediatrics 108, no. 4 (October 2001): 898–905. www.ncbi.nlm.nih.gov/pubmed/11581442/.

5. Henderson, S. T. "High Carbohydrate Diets and Alzheimer's Disease." Medical Hypotheses 62, no. 5 (2014): 689–700. doi:10.1016/j.mehy.2003.11.028. www.ncbi.nlm.nih.gov/pubmed/15082091/.

6. Neal, E.G., H. Chaffe, R. H. Schwartz, M. S. Lawson, N. Edwards, G. Fitzsimmons, A. Whitney, and J. H. Cross. "The Ketogenic Diet for the Treatment of Childhood Epilepsy: A Randomised Controlled Trial." Lancet Neurology 7, no. 6 (June 2008): 500–506. doi:10.1016/S1474-4422(08)70092-9. www.ncbi.nlm.nih.gov/pubmed/18456557.

7. Chowdhury, R., S. Warnakula, S. Kunutsor, F. Crowe, H. A. Ward, L. Johnson, et al. "Association of Dietary, Circulating, and Supplement Fatty Acids with Coronary Risk: A Systematic Review and Meta-Analysis." Annals of Internal Medicine 160 (2014): 398–406. doi:10.7326/M13-1788. annals.org/article.aspx?articleid=1846638.

8. Siri-Tarino, P. W., Q. Sun, F. B. Hu, and R. M. Krauss. "Meta-Analysis of Prospective Cohort Studies Evaluating the Association of Saturated Fat with Cardiovascular Disease." American Journal of Clinical Nutrition 91, no. 3 (March 2010): 535–46. doi:10.3945/ajcn.2009.27725. www.ncbi.nlm.nih.gov/pubmed/20071648.

9. "Prediabetes and Insulin Resistance," The National Institute of Diabetes and Digestive and Kidney Diseases. https://www.niddk.nih.gov/health-information/diabetes/types/prediabetes-insulin-resistance.

10. "National Diabetes Statistics Report," Centers for Disease Control and Prevention, 2014. http://www.cdc.gov/diabetes/pubs/statsreport14/national-diabetes-report-web.pdf.

11. Dyson, P. A., Beatty, S. and Matthews, D. R. "A low-carbohydrate diet is more effective in reducing body weight than healthy eating in both diabetic and non-diabetic subjects." Diabetic Medicine. 2007. 24: 1430–1435. http://onlinelibrary.wiley.com/doi/10.1111/j.1464-5491.2007.02290.x/full.

12. Christopher D. Gardner, PhD; Alexandre Kiazand, MD; Sofiya Alhassan, PhD; Soowon Kim, PhD; Randall S. Stafford, MD, PhD; Raymond R. Balise, PhD; Helena C. Kraemer, PhD; Abby C. King, PhD, "Comparison of the Atkins, Zone, Ornish, and LEARN Diets for Change in Weight and Related Risk Factors Among Overweight Premenopausal Women," JAMA. 2007;297(9):969-977. http://jama.jamanetwork.com/article.aspx?articleid=205916.

13. Gary D. Foster, Ph.D., Holly R. Wyatt, M.D., James O. Hill, Ph.D., Brian G. McGuckin, Ed.M., Carrie Brill, B.S., B. Selma Mohammed, M.D., Ph.D., Philippe O. Szapary, M.D., Daniel J. Rader, M.D., Joel S. Edman, D.Sc., and Samuel Klein, M.D., "A Randomized Trial of a Low-Carbohydrate Diet for Obesity – NEJM," N Engl J Med 2003; 348:2082-2090. http://www.nejm.org/doi/full/10.1056/NEJMoa022207.

14. JS Volek, MJ Sharman, AL Gómez, DA Judelson, MR Rubin, G Watson, B Sokmen, R Silvestre, DN French, and WJ Kraemer, "Comparison of Energy-restricted Very Low-carbohydrate and Low-fat Diets on Weight Loss and Body Composition in Overweight Men and Women," Nutr Metab (Lond). 2004; 1: 13. http://www.ncbi.nlm.nih.gov/pmc/articles/PMC538279/.

15. Y. Wady Aude, MD; Arthur S. Agatston, MD; Francisco Lopez-Jimenez, MD, MSc; Eric H. Lieberman, MD; Marie Almon, MS, RD; Melinda Hansen, ARNP; Gerardo Rojas, MD; Gervasio A. Lamas, MD; Charles H. Hennekens, MD, DrPH, "The National Cholesterol Education Program Diet vs a Diet Lower in Carbohydrates and Higher in Protein and Monounsaturated Fat," Arch Intern Med. 2004;164(19):2141-2146. http://archinte.jamanetwork.com/article.aspx?articleid=217514.

16. Bonnie J. Brehm, Randy J. Seeley, Stephen R. Daniels, and David A. D'Alessio, "A Randomized Trial Comparing a Very Low Carbohydrate Diet and a Calorie-Restricted Low Fat Diet on Body Weight and Cardiovascular Risk Factors in Healthy Women," The Journal of Clinical Endocrinology & Metabolism: Vol 88, No 4; January 14, 2009. http://press.endocrine.org/doi/full/10.1210/jc.2002-021480.

17. M. E. Daly, R. Paisey, R. Paisey, B. A. Millward, C. Eccles, K. Williams, S. Hammersley, K. M. MacLeod, T. J. Gale, "Short-term Effects of Severe Dietary Carbohydrate-restriction Advice in Type 2 Diabetes–a Randomized Controlled Trial," Diabetic Medicine, 2006; 23: 15–20. http://onlinelibrary.wiley.com/doi/10.1111/j.1464-5491.2005.01760.x/abstract.

18. Stephen B. Sondike, MD, Nancy Copperman, MS, RD, Marc S. Jacobson, MD, "Effects Of A Low-Carbohydrate Diet On Weight Loss And Cardiovascular Risk Factor In Overweight Adolescents," The Journal of Pediatrics: Vol 142, Issue 3: 253-258; March 2003. http://www.sciencedirect.com/science/article/pii/S0022347602402065.

19. William S. Yancy Jr., MD, MHS; Maren K. Olsen, PhD; John R. Guyton, MD; Ronna P. Bakst, RD; and Eric C. Westman, MD, MHS, "A Low-Carbohydrate, Ketogenic Diet versus a Low-Fat Diet To Treat Obesity and Hyperlipidemia: A Randomized, Controlled Trial," Ann Intern Med. 2004;140(10):769-777. http://annals.org/article.aspx?articleid=717451.

20. Grant D Brinkworth, Manny Noakes, Jonathan D Buckley, Jennifer B Keogh, and Peter M Clifton, "Long-term Effects of a Very-low-carbohydrate Weight Loss Diet Compared with an Isocaloric Low-fat Diet after 12 Mo," Am J Clin Nutr July 2009 vol. 90 no. 1 23-32. http://ajcn.nutrition.org/content/90/1/23.long.

21. H. Guldbrand, B. Dizdar, B. Bunjaku, T. Lindström, M. Bachrach-Lindström, M. Fredrikson, C. J. Östgren, F. H. Nystrom, "In Type 2 Diabetes, Randomisation to Advice to Follow a Low-carbohydrate Diet Transiently Improves Glycaemic Control Compared with Advice to Follow a Low-fat Diet Producing a Similar Weight Loss," Diabetologia (2012) 55: 2118. http://link.springer.com/article/10.1007/s00125-012-2567-4.

22. Sharon M. Nickols-Richardson, PhD, RD, , Mary Dean Coleman, PhD, RD, Joanne J. Volpe, Kathy W. Hosig, PhD, MPH, RD, "Perceived Hunger Is Lower and Weight Loss Is Greater in Overweight Premenopausal Women Consuming a Low-Carbohydrate/High-Protein vs High-Carbohydrate/Low-Fat Diet," The Journal of Pediatrics: Vol 105, Issue 9: 1433–1437; September 2005. http://www.sciencedirect.com/science/article/pii/S000282230501151X.

23. Frederick F. Samaha, M.D., Nayyar Iqbal, M.D., Prakash Seshadri, M.D., Kathryn L. Chicano, C.R.N.P., Denise A. Daily, R.D., Joyce McGrory, C.R.N.P., Terrence Williams, B.S., Monica Williams, B.S., Edward J. Gracely, Ph.D., and Linda Stern, M.D., "A Low-Carbohydrate as Compared with a Low-Fat Diet in Severe Obesity, " N Engl J Med 2003; 348:2074-2081. http://www.nejm.org/doi/full/10.1056/NEJMoa022637.

24. Yancy WS Jr, Westman EC, McDuffie JR, Grambow SC, Jeffreys AS, Bolton J, Chalecki A, Oddone EZ, "A randomized trial of a low-carbohydrate diet vs orlistat plus a low-fat diet for weight loss," Arch Intern Med. 2010 Jan 25;170(2):136-45. http://www.ncbi.nlm.nih.gov/pubmed/20101008?itool=EntrezSystem2.PEntrez.Pubmed.Pubmed_ResultsPanel.Pubmed_RVDocSum&ordinalpos=2.

25. Swasti Tiwari, Shahla Riazi, and Carolyn A. Ecelbarger, "Insulin's Impact on Renal Sodium Transport and Blood Pressure in Health, Obesity, and Diabetes," American Journal of Physiology vol. 293, no. 4 (October 2, 2007): 974–984, http://ajprenal.physiology.org/content/293/4/F974.full.

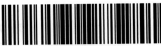

61297459R00058

Made in the USA
Middletown, DE
09 January 2018